Nurses With Disabilities

Leslie Neal-Boylan, PhD, RN, CRRN, APRN, FNP-BC, is professor and associate dean at Quinnipiac University School of Nursing in Hamden, Connecticut. She earned her BSN from Rutgers University, her MSN from San Jose State University, and her PhD in nursing from George Mason University. She received a post-master's certificate as a family nurse practitioner (FNP) from Marymount University. She is a board-certified family nurse practitioner and is also certified in rehabilitation nursing, home health nursing, and rheumatology. She also works at Care Medica Family Practice and Internal Medicine in her FNP role. Dr. Neal-Boylan has over 30 years of direct clinical experience and 15 years in nursing education. She has held various leadership positions in nursing throughout the years. She has authored and/or edited almost 100 peer-reviewed publications including seven books. Dr. Neal-Boylan's research focus has been on the nursing workforce, most recently concerning registered nurses with disabilities and retired volunteer nurses. However, she has also published on topics related to geriatric patient care, the nurse practitioner role, and chronic illness.

Nurses With Disabilities

Professional Issues and Job Retention

Leslie Neal-Boylan, PhD, RN, CRRN, APRN, FNP-BC

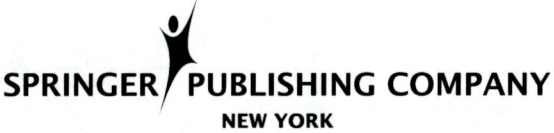

SPRINGER PUBLISHING COMPANY

NEW YORK

Copyright © 2013 Springer Publishing Company, LLC

All rights reserved.

No part of this publication may be reproduced, stored in a retrieval system, or transmitted in any form or by any means, electronic, mechanical, photocopying, recording, or otherwise, without the prior permission of Springer Publishing Company, LLC, or authorization through payment of the appropriate fees to the Copyright Clearance Center, Inc., 222 Rosewood Drive, Danvers, MA 01923, 978-750-8400, fax 978-646-8600, info@copyright.com or on the web at www.copyright.com.

Springer Publishing Company, LLC
11 West 42nd Street
New York, NY 10036
www.springerpub.com

Acquisitions Editor: Allan Graubard
Composition: diacriTech

ISBN: 978-0-8261-1010-7
E-book ISBN: 978-0-8261-1012-1

12 13 14 15 / 5 4 3 2 1

The author and the publisher of this Work have made every effort to use sources believed to be reliable to provide information that is accurate and compatible with the standards generally accepted at the time of publication. Because medical science is continually advancing, our knowledge base continues to expand. Therefore, as new information becomes available, changes in procedures become necessary. We recommend that the reader always consult current research and specific institutional policies before performing any clinical procedure. The author and publisher shall not be liable for any special, consequential, or exemplary damages resulting, in whole or in part, from the readers' use of, or reliance on, the information contained in this book. The publisher has no responsibility for the persistence or accuracy of URLs for external or third-party Internet websites referred to in this publication and does not guarantee that any content on such websites is, or will remain, accurate or appropriate.

Library of Congress Cataloging-in-Publication Data

Neal-Boylan, Leslie.
  Nurses with disabilities: professional issues and job retention / Leslie Neal-Boylan.
     p. cm.
  ISBN 978-0-8261-1010-7
  1. Nurses with disabilities. 2. Nursing. I. Title.
  RT34.N43 2012
  610.73—dc23

2012022730

Special discounts on bulk quantities of our books are available to corporations, professional associations, pharmaceutical companies, health care organizations, and other qualifying groups. If you are interested in a custom book, including chapters from more than one of our titles, we can provide that service as well.

For details, please contact:
Special Sales Department, Springer Publishing Company, LLC
11 West 42nd Street, 15th Floor, New York, NY 10036-8002
Phone: 877-687-7476 or 212-431-4370; Fax: 212-941-7842

Printed in the United States of America by Gasch Printing.

This book is dedicated to registered nurses everywhere
who devote their lives to improving
the lives of others.

To a particularly special nurse, my mother:
Natalie Rotkoff, nurse (and mother) extraordinaire!

Contents

Foreword by Geraldine Polly Bednash, PhD, RN, FAAN   ix
Foreword by Suzanne C. Smeltzer, EdD, RN, FAAN   xi
Preface   *xiii*
Acknowledgments   *xv*

1. Who Are Nurses With Disabilities?   1
2. Why Are Nurses With Disabilities Leaving Nursing?   19
3. Hiding the Disability   37
4. Disability, Job Longevity, and Career Choice   63
5. Does Having a Disability Compromise Patient Safety?   95
6. Nurses With Disabilities and the Health Care Environment   117
7. Nurse Heroics   145
8. Retaining Nurses With Disabilities   167

Appendix   *201*
Index   *205*

Foreword

The term "disability" is fraught with social and moral connotations reflecting society's belief that the disabled individual has lost significant cognitive, motor, sensory, or other functions. This perception of the term *disabled* has often led to a differentiated life or work experience for the disabled individual that is often not based on real assessment of that individual's capacity to contribute to the work of a profession, a community, or a society and can create a tremendous loss to both the individual who is disabled and our society as a whole.

This book challenges some of these preconceived notions and tells the real-world experience of nurses who have faced barriers that are not fact based and that in some cases deprived the profession or society of their capacity as fully contributing and functioning members. In the United States, and many other nations, discrimination based upon disability is outlawed. In 1990, President George W. Bush signed into law the Americans with Disabilities Act, adding disabled to the list of other protected categories in the U.S. Civil Rights Act of 1964.

The primary intent of this law was to ensure that inappropriate perceptions of an individual's capacity to be a contributing worker, professional, or member of society would not be used to limit that individual's opportunities. The law was also an example of our society's belief that in a just society, an individual should be judged by his or her contributions and work, not by appearance or perceived limitations.

This book will provide nurses with the information to make objective and fact-based assessments on this important issue. Moreover, it will arm nursing professionals with an understanding of how the issue of disability is affecting workforce supply in nursing, how accommodations can provide assistance to individuals with disabilities, and how a balanced and thoughtful approach can allow nursing professionals to function to their fullest.

Clearly, disabilities are not solely a concern for the working nursing professionals. Another, and perhaps just as important, outcome of this book will be the capacity for nurses to also understand more fully the disabled individuals for whom they provide care. The unique physical, emotional, and social needs of disabled patients will also surely be addressed more fully from this important perspective.

Geraldine Polly Bednash, PhD, RN, FAAN
Chief Executive Officer/Executive Director
American Association of Colleges of Nursing
Washington, DC

Foreword

It has been estimated that between 54 million and 60 million people in the United States live with one or more disabilities; the number exceeds 1 billion globally. Many studies have demonstrated that the health care of people with disabilities is of poorer quality than care provided to people without disabilities, and people with disabilities are less satisfied with their health care than other patient populations. Numerous physical, structural, and attitudinal barriers to obtaining quality health care have been reported by people with a variety of disabilities. As a result they receive less health care screening and primary care, and experience repeated negative encounters in their efforts to obtain appropriate health care and to receive high-quality care during hospitalization.

The U.S. Surgeon General's office issued several calls to action to improve the situation, in part by calling for inclusion of the topic of disability in educational programs for nurses, physicians, and dentists. Some efforts are underway to respond to these calls to action. Often overlooked, however, are strategies to increase the number of health care providers with disabilities by examining program admissions criteria, opening admissions procedures to qualified candidates with disabilities, and undertaking strategies that allow health care professionals who acquire disabilities as adults to continue their work in health care. They are often not provided with the accommodations that are mandated by the Americans with Disabilities Act of 1990 that would enable them to continue their contributions to their profession and to patient care. As a result, many health care professionals with disabilities end up leaving the work setting and often their profession, even when the need for providers with expertise is growing and a shortage of experienced health care professionals is acute.

Fearing discrimination and other negative reactions from their employers, coworkers, and peers, some health care providers with disabilities hide their disabilities, depriving them of accommodations that could make their work easier and allow them to continue working. This also deprives the profession, employers, and patients of the expertise of nurses who could have a major impact on the care of patients, including those with disabilities.

Despite the call to integrate disability-related content and issues in the education of health professionals, the profession and educational programs have been slow to respond. Although faculty in health professions education have been encouraged to develop and implement strategies to improve preparation of their students for caring for patients with disabilities, there has been little attention to what people with disabilities who are students in the health care professions bring to the educational setting. In addition to joining the ranks of health care professions, their presence in the classroom and clinical environment can change the negative attitudes and stereotypes held by other students and faculty as well as society as a whole. Further, they can utilize their own personal experiences and views as a person with a disability to improve the care given to patients with disabilities.

Nurses With Disabilities: Professional Issues and Job Retention has brought together information and real-life experiences of nurses who have disabilities. It will serve as an invaluable source of information on the impact of disability on the employment and retention of registered nurses.

Suzanne C. Smeltzer, EdD, RN, FAAN
Professor and Director, Center for Nursing Research
Villanova University College of Nursing
Villanova, PA

Preface

I first learned of the scarcity of literature regarding nurses with disabilities when a graduate student of mine mentioned that she had come across a lot of work on students with disabilities but none on nurses. This was several years ago and I didn't pursue doing anything about it until the idea had germinated for a while. When my close friend and colleague, Dr. Sharron Guillett, and I decided to explore the experiences of nurses with disabilities, we asked the student if she would like to be included. She declined and wished us luck in exploring this new territory.

Sharron and I were fascinated with the topic: Sharron, because she has a family member with a disability, and I because of my work as a rehabilitation nurse. As we talked to nurses with disabilities we learned how our supposedly compassionate profession had mostly turned its back on these nurses. Although invaluable work has been done about the experiences of student nurses with disabilities, when we sought collaboration on our work about nurses with disabilities, to our amazement we were refused because Sharron and I were not disabled. The perspective was that we had no right or ability to shed light on the experiences of nurses with disabilities if we were not, ourselves, disabled.

Neither of us ever claimed to know what it was like to be personally disabled but we did know about caring for people with disabilities and we did know that someone had to bring their experiences to light. But this book is much more than the four research studies that buttress it. It was also informed by the many nurses who have come up to us at conferences and otherwise shared their stories, so similar in experience and outcome to those of our research participants. It has become clear, over time, that the issues nurses with disabilities face are serious and irredeemable unless we decide to act.

The experience of being a nurse with a disability, according to the voices of these nurses, exemplifies the experience of anyone with a disability who is trying to work without discrimination. It also exemplifies the experience of simply being a nurse in this day and age because, as nurses, we often sacrifice ourselves physically and mentally in the course of doing our jobs. Chapter 7, "Nurse Heroics," discusses how the expectation of nurses is to work above and beyond regardless of our own health and well-being. We tend to look down on nurses who are not willing to miss breaks, meals, and days off in service to the profession. I say "in service to the profession" and not "in service to our patients" because we don't do our patients any favors by being angry and resentful or sick and tired when we are at work. We also don't benefit them when we don't role model all of the healthful behaviors we preach to them.

The intention of this book is not to scold but to present the issues facing nurses with disabilities using their own voices and to attempt to offer potential solutions. Chapter 1 lays a foundation by introducing to or reminding the reader about legislation that affects persons with disabilities and by briefly describing the research studies that ground the book. Chapter 2 describes why nurses with disabilities are leaving nursing. Chapter 3 continues the dialogue by discussing the interesting phenomenon of many nurses with disabilities attempting to hide their disabilities and the perspectives of nurse recruiters and managers regarding hiring nurses with disabilities.

Job longevity and career decisions are analyzed in Chapter 4. Nurses with disabilities often leave the profession, sometimes of their own accord, but more often because they feel pushed out. How do they decide to leave and what do they do next? Chapter 4 addresses these questions.

Chapter 5 explores the common perception that nurses with disabilities jeopardize patient safety. There are no data to support this perception, yet it is pervasive. Nurses are trained to think scientifically yet that is not demonstrated in this case.

Chapter 6 illustrates how the nurse with a disability interacts within his or her environment with colleagues, administrators, and patients. Nurse testimonials describe how these interactions affect the work life of these nurses. Managers and patients lend their voices as well to this discussion.

Following Chapter 7, "Nurse Heroics," Chapter 8 attempts to provide solutions to the issues presented throughout the book. Specific suggestions are given for altering the way we educate nurses and what nurse educators and clinicians with disabilities should consider as they plan their careers. Nurse leaders and administrators are advised about specific approaches they can use to minimize the hemorrhage of nurses with disabilities from the profession.

I hope readers will see that as many perspectives as possible were presented in the writing of this book. Furthermore, many of the experiences described were positive and serve to further illustrate that we can approach the issues in positive ways and that it is possible to be open minded, compassionate, and creative when necessary to support our colleagues, whether or not they are disabled.

Acknowledgments

I'd like to thank my beloved friend and colleague, Dr. Sharron E. Guillett, for her work regarding nurses with disabilities. I admire her for her keen intelligence, incredible strength, and dedication to nursing and nurses.

I also want to thank my husband for his enduring love, support, and editing assistance while writing this book.

Most importantly, I am supremely grateful to all of the nurses who shared their stories and experiences with me and had faith that by exposing the issues that they live with day to day, the profession might make changes that would benefit all of us.

Finally, I'd like to sincerely thank every nurse who reads this book through, because in doing so you show that you are willing to hear about the sometimes ugly side of our beloved profession, and awareness is the first step toward meaningful change.

1

Who Are Nurses With Disabilities?

Sue is a 54-year-old registered nurse with 30 years of nursing experience. She has always been a hard worker and she has extensive expertise and experience as a critical care nurse. She has always prided herself on being able to care for her patients without needing to ask her colleagues for help, except in extreme situations. Sue was diagnosed with rheumatoid arthritis 5 years ago but never mentioned this to her supervisor or colleagues. However, in the past year, she began to feel very fatigued and in frequent pain. She found herself asking other staff to help her with tasks she could previously manage on her own. She has also been using her sick leave and taking more time off than she has ever taken before. Her manager suggested that Sue might not be capable of doing this kind of work anymore and asked if it might not be best for her to leave critical care and work in another area of nursing. Sue was shocked and dismayed to hear her manager speak to her this way and assured her that she could do the work and that she wanted to stay on the unit. Sue found her own ways of compensating for what she could no longer easily do but sensed that her colleagues did not approve of her compensatory techniques even though they worked well and did not compromise patient safety. Not long after this, Sue had her annual review. Despite having had excellent reviews every year, this review indicated that her manager was not pleased with her work. Sue decided to leave the job. Sue was not given any information by the manager or by a Human Resources representative regarding her disability rights before she left. Nor was she given any specific options for working in another area of the facility in order to stay there.

Registered nurses with disabilities appear to be facing discrimination of one form or another in the work place. This discrimination is occasionally blatant but more often masked by disapproval of how the nurse is performing even if the care he or she is providing does not differ significantly from the care the nurse has always provided. Nurses with disabilities tend to leave nursing or find jobs that are not physically demanding or they go back to school to move further from the bedside. These nurses have expertise and are often very experienced. They tend to love nursing and they grieve when they cannot continue to be part of the profession. The profession has undergone many shortages as it ebbs and flows from decade to decade. It is important to the profession to try to understand why nurses with disabilities often perceive themselves as being pushed out of the profession and what can be done to retain them.

To date, several research studies have been done to explore the work life experiences of nurses with disabilities, to learn who these nurses are, the settings in which they work, and their successes and struggles. This chapter explores the data about people with disabilities, in general, and about nurses with disabilities, in particular. This will set the stage for the rest of the book as it explores the work life experiences of nurses with disabilities.

BACKGROUND

It is currently unknown how many registered nurses have physical and/or sensory disabilities. However, according to the most recent data from the Census Bureau which gets its data from the American Community Survey (ACS), approximately 41 million nonmilitary, noninstitutionalized people in the United States considered themselves disabled in 2006. Of these people, approximately 4% had a sensory disability (hearing, vision, or communication) and 9% had a physical disability. Of those 16 years old or older, 7% described themselves as having an employment disability. Within the working age population (16 years to 64 years), 12% reported having a disability.

The rate of disability increases to almost 16% of the total population when people in the military and those living in group homes, whether institutional or in the community, are included (Brault, 2008; U.S. Census Bureau, 2006a, 2006b). The Centers for Disease Control and Prevention (CDC) estimates that 71.4 million people in the United States have disabilities (CDC, 2011; www.cdc.gov/nchs/fastats/disable.htm). Approximately 16 million of these have problems with mobility, 35 million have trouble hearing, and 19 million have difficulty with vision (CDC, 2011).

DEFINING DISABILITY

There are many definitions of disability. The Americans with Disabilities Act (ADA) of 1990 (Public Law 101-336) defines disability as "with respect to an individual, a physical or mental impairment that substantially limits one or more of the major life activities of such individual; a record of such an impairment; or being regarded as having such an impairment.

The phrase "physical or mental impairment" means—

- Any physiological disorder or condition, cosmetic disfigurement, or anatomical loss affecting one or more of the following body systems: neurological; musculoskeletal; special sense organs; respiratory, including speech organs; cardiovascular; reproductive; digestive; genitourinary; hemic and lymphatic; skin; and endocrine
- Any mental or psychological disorder such as mental retardation, organic brain syndrome, emotional or mental illness, and specific learning disabilities
- The phrase physical or mental impairment includes, but is not limited to, such contagious and noncontagious diseases and conditions as orthopedic, visual, speech, and hearing impairments; cerebral palsy; epilepsy; muscular dystrophy; multiple sclerosis; cancer; heart disease; diabetes; mental retardation; emotional illness; specific learning disabilities; HIV disease (whether symptomatic or asymptomatic); tuberculosis; drug addiction; and alcoholism (http://www.ada.gov/regs2010/titleIII_2010/titleIII_2010_regulations.htm#a104)

This definition supports the concept of a chronic illness as a disability. Such has been the case with many of the nurses studied who self-identified as having a disability. The research on which this book is based did not include nurses with cognitive or behavioral disabilities.

The World Health Organization (WHO) states that:

> Disabilities is an umbrella term, covering impairments, activity limitations, and participation restrictions. An impairment is a problem in body function or structure; an activity limitation is a difficulty encountered by an individual in executing a task or action; while a participation restriction is a problem experienced by an individual in involvement in life situations. (http://www.who.int/topics/disabilities/en)

This definition applies to a discussion of nurses with disabilities because they may have self-imposed restrictions or restrictions imposed or suggested by others related to their work. Many of the nurses studied found safe ways to compensate for what they could no longer do in the traditional way, so according to the WHO definition, they would not be viewed as having an activity restriction. Despite this, colleagues and administrators do not always support compensatory methods and therefore may make it appear as if the nurse has an activity limitation.

The United States Equal Employment Opportunity Commission's (EEOC) definition of disability is a physical condition that significantly limits one or more major life activities, such as seeing or walking. A history of disability may allow the person to be considered disabled if the person has an impairment (mental or physical) that is expected to last more than 6 months. In other words, this qualifies someone who has a medical condition that may cause disability to be considered disabled, even if they don't currently have the disability.

The definition of disability that is used will ultimately impact how issues regarding disability are approached and viewed (Neal-Boylan, in press). What one person may view as a disability, another may not view as a disability. To retain nurses with disabilities, it is important that nursing not define disability in such a way as to be used as an excuse to push out a nurse who is simply not wanted in the setting for other reasons.

The ADA does not permit prospective employers to ask applicants questions about the disability before offering the job. Employers are required to make "reasonable accommodation" to "otherwise qualified individuals . . . unless it results in undue hardship." According to the ADA, the prospective employer must be aware of the disability in order to respect the rights of the person with disabilities. This seems self-evident. However, as will be explained later in this book, nurses often feel the need to hide their disabilities in order to obtain employment in nursing (http://www.ada.gov/cguide.htm#anchor62335).

For the purposes of the research studies upon which this book is based, the nurses involved self-identified as having a physical and/or sensory disability. The nurses often discussed the handicapping aspects of their disabilities. It is important to distinguish a disability from a handicap. Someone may have a disability but because they can compensate in some form or another, or in cases when they are doing something that has no relevance to whether or not they have a disability, they would not be considered handicapped. The disability contributes to a handicap when the person is unable to perform a task or do something they might otherwise do because they have a disability. However, anyone, whether or not they have an identified disability, might be judged as conceivably having a handicap depending on the situation. A student who has stayed up all night partying instead of studying, for instance, might be handicapped by lack of sleep and might be unable to take the test to the best of his or her ability if the student had gotten a full night's sleep.

For the purposes of this book, disability is defined the way the nurses in the research studies defined it. Nurses who participated in the research studies on which this book is largely based self-identified as having chronic illnesses, severe allergies, difficulties with mobility, sensory impairments, and many "hidden disabilities." Many nurses who participated had multiple disabilities. Table 1.1 includes the various disabilities self-identified by nurses in these studies.

It is important to note that nurses may have cognitive or emotional disabilities that can significantly impact nursing work. The research on which this book is based specifically excluded nurses who self-identified as having cognitive or emotional disabilities except when one of these occurred concomitantly with a physical and/or sensory disability. This decision was made because it is very hard to distinguish whether the way in which a nurse perceives he or she is treated on the job is directly attributed to the disability or is because the nurse is angry or cognitively impaired. In the course of the research, the author received several phone calls from nurses who said they wanted to participate and reported that they had cognitive or emotional disabilities. These nurses tended to sound very angry and it was hard to elicit specific details of their experiences. Clearly, this is a population that should also be studied as it is probable that these nurses have been the recipients of discriminatory practices. Their voices should also be heard. However, doing so was not within the scope of the studies that were done and therefore the experience of having a cognitive or emotional disability will not be discussed in this book.

TABLE 1.1
Self-Identified Disabilities

Rheumatoid arthritis	Joint pain
Back pain	Epilepsy or other seizure disorder
Crohn's disease	Post polio syndrome
Osteoarthritis	Spinal cord injury
Herniated disc	Multiple sclerosis
Psoriatic arthritis	Latex allergy
Hearing impairment	Stroke
Status post brain tumor	Diabetes mellitus
Fibromyalgia	Muscular dystrophy
Fused wrist/foot	Visual impairment
Tetralogy of Fallot	Speech disorder
Ureterostomy	Wrist joint removal
Deafness	Missing joints
Paraplegia	Amputation
Chronic pain	

EMPLOYMENT

According to the U.S. Department of Labor, Bureau of Labor Statistics (2012; http://www.bls.gov/news.release/empsit.t06.htm), as of October 2011 the number of civilian, noninstitutionalized people aged 16 years and older with disabilities who were employed was 5,037 (in thousands) out of 27,214 (in thousands) as opposed to 135,949 (in thousands) out of 213,055 (in thousands) of those not disabled. This demonstrates that while approximately a quarter of people with disabilities are employed, closer to half of those without disabilities are employed. The unemployment rate for those with disabilities was approximately 13%, which is a slight decrease from the year before and is approximately 8% which is largely the same as the year before for those without disabilities. The unemployment rate for women with disabilities was slightly lower than that for men with disabilities. These data included people with cognitive, sensory, and physical disabilities.

People with disabilities are often self-employed as compared to people without disabilities and are more likely than those without disabilities to work part time. People with disabilities are less likely than those without a disability to work in professional or management jobs (Bureau of Labor Statistics/news.release/disabl.nr0.htm). It costs the United States government approximately $232 billion every year to support employable adults with disabilities who are not employed (Office on Disability Prevalence and Impact fact sheet; http://www.hhs.gov/od/about/fact_sheets/prevalenceandimpact.html).

Impairments in physical function increase as one ages. The number of people with disabilities is significantly higher for adults aged 65 years and older than for younger populations (Brault, 2008). As the population of nurses age, it is expected that those with functional impairments will increase (Bristo, Ciotti, McCulloh, Lyons, & Carroll, 2005; Neal-Boylan, 2012; Wray, Aspland, Gibson, Stimpson, & Watson, 2009). Older nurses may find that the physical aspect of nursing becomes more difficult with age (Mion et al., 2006; O'Brien-Pallas, Duffield, & Alksnis, 2004). Aging nurses are needed to remain in nursing as they have experience (Fitzgerald, 2007) and can mentor younger nurses as well as strengthen the nursing workforce during times of shortage (Cocca-Bates & Neal-Boylan, 2011). This fact that nurses are aging and are sought after to remain in the nursing workforce further validates the need to learn how to retain nurses with disabilities in nursing.

As one 67-year-old nurse said:

> I realize that I can't be lugging patients around. . . . It is the realization that I have my limits and the expectation that really all nurses have health limits for lifting patients. I have to speak up and let

them know what my limits are and how I'm going to accommodate my limits and how I'm going to accommodate the unit and safety.

DISABILITY BENEFITS

Interestingly, not all of the nurses studied knew about or applied for disability benefits from their workplace or sought legal counsel to try to get any benefits or accommodations for which they were eligible. It is worth reviewing what legal options may be open to nurses with disabilities if they choose to access them.

The Social Security Administration states that persons eligible for disability benefits have a medical problem that will last at least one year or could result in death. Their definition does not include short-term disability or partial disability. A "recent work test" and a "duration of work" test are necessary to meet the Social Security Administration's strict guidelines for receiving disability benefits (http://www.ssa.gov/pubs/10029.html).

There are also short-term disability benefits that one can obtain through their work. Depending on the employer, the employee may need to use up all sick days before the employee can access short-term disability benefits. Typically the employee needs to have worked for the employer for a specified period of time before they have access to this benefit and they have to work near full time (30 hours) or full time. Typically the employer pays the benefit but states differ regarding whether employers are required to offer this benefit. The percentage of pay and the length of time the employee may receive disability pay vary depending on the plan (http://employeebenefits.about.com/od/ancillaryinsurance/a/STDBasics.htm).

The Family and Medical Leave Act (FMLA) allows employees to take unpaid leave from work for a medical condition or a family reason. A medical condition that is serious enough to render the employee "unable to perform the essential functions" of the job is one of the requirements that makes someone eligible to receive FMLA. The Act allows for 12 weeks off within 12 months and includes job and insurance protection during that period. The employee must receive medical certification that they are eligible for FMLA (http://www.dol.gov/whd/fmla/USDeptofLabor).

Many nurses seem reluctant to apply for or request these benefits. This may be because they feel they should work through their pain or disability (see Chapter 7) or they may not see themselves as disabled and therefore eligible for these benefits. Others may think that acquiring these benefits may stigmatize them or effect their future work opportunities. It is important that employers make sure that nurses are not only aware of the options if they are disabled or ill or become so, but that they clearly understand them.

DISCRIMINATION

The Rehabilitation Act of 1973 (Americans with Disabilities Act, 2005) prohibits employers who receive federal monies, work within federal agencies, or hire federal contractors from discriminating against anyone because of their disability (http://www.ada.gov/cguide.htm#anchor65610).

According to the EEOC, if an employee is treated in a way that violates the ADA or the Rehabilitation Act (1973), then they have suffered disability discrimination. According to these laws, persons with disabilities (this includes a history of disability or chronic illness) must be provided with "reasonable accommodation."

> A reasonable accommodation is any change in the work environment (or in the way things are usually done) to help a person with a disability apply for a job, perform the duties of a job, or enjoy the benefits and privileges of employment. (http://www.eeoc.gov/laws/types/disability.cfm)

The law requires that access be provided (such as with wheelchairs) and that assistance in some cases (such as for someone who is blind) be offered. The employer is not expected to have to undergo "undue hardship" or expense to provide reasonable accommodation. According to the EEOC:

> Undue hardship means that the accommodation would be too difficult or too expensive to provide, in light of the employer's size, financial resources, and the needs of the business. An employer may not refuse to provide an accommodation just because it involves some cost. An employer does not have to provide the exact accommodation the employee or job applicant wants. If more than one accommodation works, the employer may choose which one to provide.

It is also unlawful to discriminate against people because they are related to someone who has a disability. People with disabilities must not suffer discrimination in the hiring or firing processes through pay, jobs to which they are assigned, promotions, or in anything else related to their employment. It is also unlawful to harass anyone with a disability or who once had a disability. Offensive comments that pertain to the disability and remarks that serve to foster a work environment that is hostile to the person with the disability are illegal. Supervisors, coworkers, and clients are all subject to this law.

Interestingly, nurses applying for a job cannot, by law, be asked medical questions or be required to take a physical examination before the job offer is made. They may not be asked about their disability or the extent of the disability. However, one can ask the nurse if he or she can do the job whether or not there are accommodations. If the nurse is offered the job and has the medical exam, the employer may decide to make the job conditional on certain health-related questions or the passing of the medical exam as long as all employees new to that same type of job are required to do the same. After the nurse has started in the job, medical questions and a medical exam are allowed only if documentation is needed to support accommodation or it is perceived that the nurse cannot do the job safely or effectively (http://www.eeoc.gov/laws/types/disability.cfm).

NURSES WITH DISABILITIES

Despite the higher incidence of disability in older adults, nurses of all adult ages have disabilities. Nurses with disabilities work in all settings both community and institution based. However, they appear to be least likely to remain in the hospital. Perhaps this is because hospital work tends to be very demanding physically. Interestingly, difficulty hearing in hospital nurses is associated with an increased risk of leaving the job when compared with nurses with hearing disabilities who work outside of the hospital (Neal-Boylan, Fennie, & Baldauf-Wagner, 2011). Table 1.2 lists work settings of the nurses with disabilities who were studied. However, this is by no means a complete list of settings in which nurses with disabilities work.

TABLE 1.2
Settings and Jobs in Which Nurses With Disabilities Practice

Dialysis center/clinic	Skilled nursing facility
Insurance company	Medical-surgical nursing
Legal nurse consultant	Occupational health
Nurse manager (telephonically)	Orthopedics
Pregnancy care clinic/maternal child health unit	Home care
	Office nursing
Private practice	Rehabilitation
Psychiatric/mental health	Gerontology
Public health	Education
School	Oncology
Surgery center	Prison nursing
Telephonic diseases management	Informatics
Online education	Pediatric primary care
Emergency, oncology center	Professional membership organization
Hospice	Day surgery
Women's health	Intensive care unit (ICU)
Travel nursing	Nurse anesthesia
	Health counseling

Nurses may begin their careers in any setting that utilizes nurses. However, once the disability is acquired or once it begins to cause a handicap to the nurse at work, nurses are often made to feel that they are no longer fit to work in that setting or the nurses themselves may choose to leave that setting. Nurses may leave because they fear they will jeopardize patient safety or because they feel that the compensatory techniques they use to do their jobs are not sufficient in their view or in others'. Frequently, fatigue, reduced stamina, and the inability to float to other units or to work nights or 12-hour shifts interfere with the ability to remain in the job.

When nurses leave an inpatient position, for instance, they may go back to school to prepare them for a position that will move them further away from physical care or a position that requires or puts less emphasis on the need to do physical work. This is an important distinction as job descriptions don't always match the work of the job and while the expectation may be for physical labor such as lifting patients, the nurse often has assistance from nurses' aides and others to perform the physical work. Infrequently, the organization for which the nurse works will assist the nurse to remain in the facility in a different position, thereby retaining a loyal and valuable employee.

Nurses who leave a position they love or leave the profession tend to grieve the loss and search for ways to remain in nursing despite the disability. Interestingly, they are not as likely as one might suppose to pursue disability benefits or to lodge formal complaints about discrimination. In a study of physicians with disabilities, this was also found to be true (Neal-Boylan et al., 2012)

Many nurses come to nursing with disabilities but more appear likely to acquire a disability once they become nurses. This is easily explained by the fact that most nursing schools are still reluctant to permit students with disabilities that affect physical functioning to either be admitted or to remain in school. There appears to be a common traditional belief that nursing students must be able to engage in the physical labor of caring for patients in order to become nurses. This is counterintuitive to the image that nursing is eager to portray; that is, a profession that should be valued for critical thinking and the ability to make sound and decisive judgments that direct patient care. In addition, many nurses acquire disabilities after they begin working either from injuries suffered on the job, such as back injuries, or from aging. Life in general contributes to some injuries. Further, some chronic illnesses that may not initially cause functional disability may do so as one ages or as one is exposed to a job, such as nursing, that may require physical labor, long work hours, and stamina.

Both male and female nurses have disabilities, although women have been more likely to participate in the research studies on nurses with disabilities than men. In addition, female nurses still outnumber male nurses, in general. Nurses who participated in the studies ranged in age from 26 to 77 years. Many of these were working when they participated in the research. Others were not working because they left nursing for reasons related to their disabilities. Recruiting nurses with disabilities to participate in research studies is not hard. However, finding nurses with disabilities who are still working as nurses is.

THE RESEARCH

This book is based upon four research studies and several anecdotal encounters with nurses with disabilities. All of the studies were grounded by a conceptual framework, "the integrative model of health care working conditions on organizational climate and safety" (Stone et al., 2005) (see Figure 1.1).

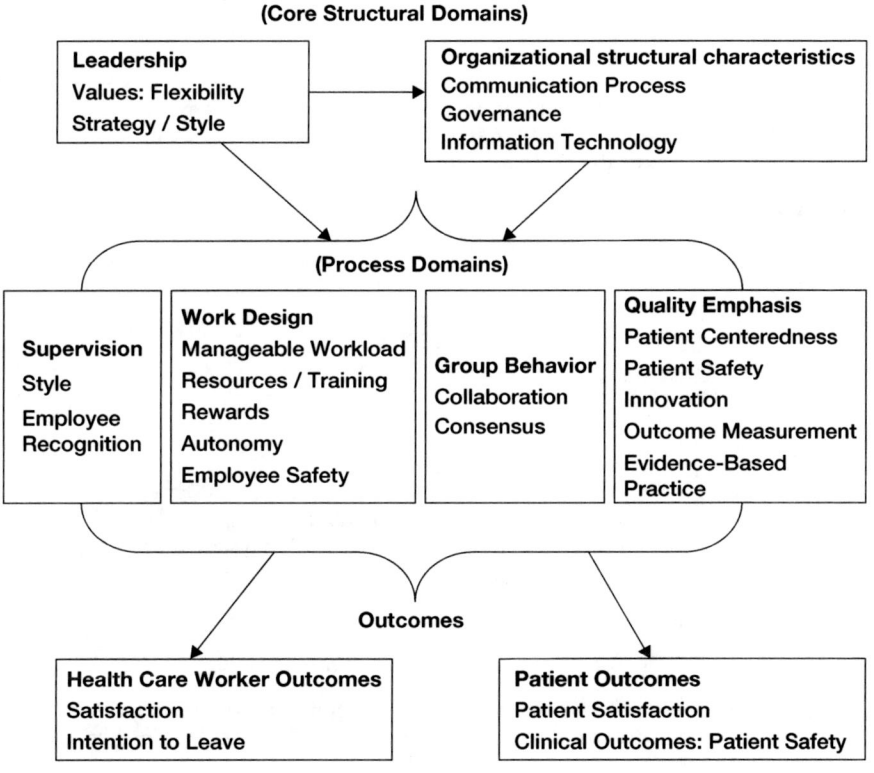

FIGURE 1.1
An integrative model of the relationships between health care working conditions and organizational climate and safety.

The first study (Guillett, Neal-Boylan, & Lathrop, 2007; Neal-Boylan & Guillett, 2008a, 2008b, 2008c) included 10 registered nurses who self-identified as having a physical and/or sensory disability and 10 nurse recruiters/managers. The study was done in Maine, Washington, DC, and Virginia. The nurses were interviewed using rigorous qualitative research methods, the data were transcribed verbatim and then analyzed. Table 1.3 lists the research questions that guided the first study and Table 1.4 includes the unstructured interview guide that was used to explore the experience of having a disability.

The second study (Neal-Boylan, Fennie, & Baldauf-Wagner, 2011) sought to focus on nurses with sensory disabilities: hearing communication and/or visual disabilities. Working nurses were sought but it soon became clear that many nurses with disabilities are not working. Nurses with visual problems who were able to accommodate by wearing glasses did not perceive themselves as being disabled. The majority of participants

TABLE 1.3
Research Questions Research Study #1

How does the work of an RN change once he/she becomes disabled?
Does his/her perception of nursing change once the RN becomes disabled?
What are the barriers to the profession for the RN with disabilities?
What are the facilitators to the profession once the RN becomes disabled?
What modifications could be made to the profession to enhance the ability of the RN with disabilities to participate in the nursing profession?

TABLE 1.4
Unstructured Interview Guide Research Study #1

For the RN with a disability

In what way do you consider yourself to be disabled?
How has your condition influenced your ability to practice as an RN?
Has having a disability changed the way you feel about nursing?
What, if any, barriers do you see to practice as an RN with a disability?
What, if any, facilitators do you see to practice as an RN?
Tell me about them.
What could be done to facilitate practice for RNs with disabilities?

For the nurse who hires other nurses

Do you hire or have you hired RNs with physical disabilities? Tell me about that.
Are there conditions that would affect an RNs ability to practice if he/she had a disability?
What would be a condition that might limit their practice?
Do you see barriers? Facilitators?
What does and could your organization do to reduce the barriers, if there are any?

had hearing disabilities. However, there were some participants with visual and communication disabilities. This study used the United States Census Questions on Disability (Table 1.5) to determine if someone had a sensory disability and the extent of that disability. Nurses were surveyed using the Nurse Work Instability Scale (Nurse WIS; Gilworth et al., 2007), which measured the risk of leaving the job. The tool was originally designed for nurses with musculoskeletal impairments but this study also evaluated its reliability with nurses with sensory disabilities and most of the questions were found to be reliable. Table 1.6 includes the research aims for this study.

The third research study (Neal-Boylan, 2012; Neal-Boylan et al., 2012) explored and compared the work life experiences of nurses and physicians with self-identified physical and/or sensory disabilities. Ten RNs and

TABLE 1.5

Census Questions on Disability Research Study #2

The next questions ask about difficulties you may have doing certain activities because of a health problem.
1. Do you have difficulty seeing, even if wearing glasses?
   a. No – no difficulty
   b. Yes – some difficulty
   c. Yes – a lot of difficulty
   d. Cannot do at all
2. Do you have difficulty hearing, even if using a hearing aid?
   a. No – no difficulty
   b. Yes – some difficulty
   c. Yes – a lot of difficulty
   d. Cannot do at all
3. Using your usual (customary) language, do you have difficulty communicating, for example, understanding or being understood?
   a. No – no difficulty
   b. Yes – some difficulty
   c. Yes – a lot of difficulty
   d. Cannot do at all

Source: www.census.gov/prod/2006pubs/p70-107.pdf

TABLE 1.6

Research Aims for Research Study #2

To determine the demographic characteristics of RNs with hearing, visual, or communication disabilities.
To explore work instability and the risk of job retention problems among nurses with sensory disabilities.
To determine whether the Nurse Work Instability Scale (Nurse-WIS) is a reliable tool to measure work instability in nurses with hearing, visual, or communication disabilities.

10 physicians were interviewed. The nurses were interviewed (Table 1.7) by a nurse and the physicians were interviewed by a physician. The coding team that analyzed the results consisted of three nurses, one of whom was disabled, and two physicians, one of whom was also disabled. Interestingly, physicians and nurses with disabilities had very similar work-life experiences. The research questions that framed the study are in Table 1.8.

The fourth study (Table 1.9) explored the match or mismatch between nurse job descriptions and the actual work of the job for registered nurses with disabilities. A purposive, theoretical sample of RNs from throughout the United States was sought. Seventeen nurses were interviewed and the interviews were transcribed verbatim. The idea for this study arose out of the previous findings that many nurses with disabilities felt discriminated against due to the perception that they were not performing their jobs as they should be. The question then arose as to whether nurses were always provided with job descriptions when they were hired and then whether the actual work they did was aligned with what was proscribed in the job descriptions. If nurses were hired with the idea that they would lift

TABLE 1.7
Unstructured Interview Guide Research Study #3

In what way do you consider yourself to be disabled? Or could you describe your disability?
How has your condition influenced your ability to practice as a physician/RN if at all?
Have you needed to compensate for your disability in any way?
How has/does your disability influence interactions at work, if at all? With patients? With colleagues?
What, if any, barriers do you see to practice as a physician/RN with a disability?
What, if any, facilitators do you see to practice as a physician/RN with a disability?
Given your disability, what organizational (or professional) changes would facilitate your ability to practice successfully?
How has your disability influenced your career choices to date? How might it influence future career choices?
Have you experienced discrimination because of your disability?

TABLE 1.8
Research Questions Research Study #3

What is it like to be a physician/RN with a physical disability?
How does the work change, if at all, in light of the physical disability?
What barriers does the physical disability present to the physician/RN with a disability?
How does the physical disability influence career decisions of the physician/RN?
Does the disability jeopardize the ability of the physician/RN to practice medicine/nursing safely?
How do the experiences of the RNS and physicians compare with regard to having a physical disability?

TABLE 1.9
Research Questions and Unstructured Interview Guide for Research Study #4

1. How is the description of nurse responsibilities managed during the hiring interview?
2. In actuality, what is the experience of the nurse with regard to fulfilling all of the duties listed in the job description?
3. If the nurse's disability impacts the nurse's ability to perform the work, then what is the experience of the nurse regarding the need to compensate in order to fulfill her/his responsibilities?
4. What are the perceptions of the nurse regarding the outcomes/responses of others to the nurse's inability to perform a skill/task or the nurse's attempts to compensate?

and move patients and do other very physical activities, then it would be reasonable to assume that they should be able to do these things while they were working. However, if physical activity with patients was not included in their original job descriptions, then how could they be pushed out of their jobs for not being able to perform those activities? Interestingly, the nurses who were recruited for this study were working in areas that they sought out and that were willing, for the most part, to accommodate them.

Overall, while doing the research, it was a challenge to find nurses with disabilities who either felt comfortable and accommodated in their work (if they did, they typically had sought that work themselves or were employed by others with disabilities) or who were working as nurses at all. The profession should want to recruit and retain nurses who think well and who can contribute their intelligence to the profession and, as well, should seek to practice what it preaches to patients by seeking ways to use nurses with disabilities in some form or capacity. This book hopes to make that possible.

It is interesting to examine the comments and experiences of the nurses who participated in the research studies and of nurses who have anecdotally contributed their comments regarding their experiences at work. In light of the laws regarding the prevention of discrimination and the necessity for reasonable accommodation, it is confusing and disheartening that many nurses with disabilities have expressed that they were not met with lawful responses to the challenges they faced in the workplace.

It is clear that Sue, the nurse described in the case at the beginning of the chapter, is only one example of a nurse who feels pushed out of the job and does not know where to turn to be able to remain in nursing. The purpose of this book is to enlighten readers regarding the experience of these nurses and to suggest ways we can retain nurses with disabilities and not deter them from staying in nursing either from outright discriminatory practices or from ignorance of what a person with a disability can bring to their work.

REFERENCES

Americans with Disabilities Act. (2005). *Disability rights section: A guide to disability rights laws*. U.S. Department of Justice Civil Rights Division. Retrieved from http://www.ada.gov/cguide.htm#anchor65610

Brault, M. W. (2008). Americans with disabilities 2005: Household economic studies. *Current Population Reports*, pp. 70–117. Retrieved from http://www.census.gov/prod/2008pubs/p70-117.pdf

Bristo, M., Ciotti, R., McCulloh, K., Lyons, K., & Carroll, S. (2005). Disabilities don't stop these nurses. Interview by Barbara Weiss. *RN, 68*(1), 45–46, 48.

Bureau of Labor Statistics. (2012). *Persons with a disability: Labor force characteristics Summary*. Retrieved from http://www.bls.gov/news.release/disabl.nr0.htm

Centers for Disease Control. (2011). *Disability and functioning (adults)*. Retrieved from www.cdc.gov/nchs/fastats/disable.htm

Cocca, K., & Neal-Boylan, L. J. (2011). Retired RNs: Perceptions of volunteering. *Geriatric Nursing, 32*(2), 96–105.

Fitzgerald, D. C. (2007). Aging, experienced nurses: Their value and needs. *Contemporary Nurse, 24*(2), 237–42.

Gilworth, G., Bhakta, B., Eyres, S., Carey, A., Chamberlain, M. A., & Tennant, A. (2007). Keeping nurses working: Development and psychometric testing of the Nurse-Work-Instability Scale (NURSE-WIS). *Journal of Advanced Nursing, 57*(5), 543–551.

Guillett, S. E., Neal-Boylan, L. J., & Lathrop, R. (2007). Ready, willing, and disabled. *American Nurse Today, 2*(8), 30–32.

Mion, L. C., Hazel, C., Cap, M., Fusilero, J., Podmore, M. L., & Szweda, C. (2006). Retaining and recruiting mature experienced nurses: A multicomponent organizational strategy. *Journal of Nursing Administration, 36*(3), 148–154.

Neal-Boylan, L. J. (2012). An exploration and comparison of the worklife experiences of registered nurses and physicians with permanent physical and/or sensory disabilities. *Rehabilitation Nursing, 37*(1), 3–10.

Neal-Boylan, L. (in press). Rehabilitation clients in the community. In F. A. Maurer & C. M. Smith (Eds.), *Community/public health nursing practice: Health for families and populations* (5th ed.).

Neal-Boylan, L., Fennie, K., & Baldauf-Wagner, S. (2011). Nurses with sensory disabilities: Their perceptions and characteristics. *Rehabilitation Nursing, 36*(1), 25–31.

Neal-Boylan, L., & Guillett, S. E. (2008a). Registered nurses with physical disabilities. *Journal of Nursing Administration, 38*(1), 1–3.

Neal-Boylan, L., & Guillett, S. E. (2008b). Work experiences of RNs with physical disabilities. *Rehabilitation Nursing, 33*(2), 67–72.

Neal-Boylan, L. J., & Guillett, S. E. (2008c). Nurses with disabilities: Can changing our educational system keep them in nursing? *Nurse Educator, 33*(4), 1–4.

Neal-Boylan, L., Hopkins, A., Skeete, R., Hartmann, S. B., Iezzoni, L. I., & Nunez-Smith, M. (2012). The career trajectories of health care professionals practicing with permanent disabilities. *Academic Medicine, 87*(2), 172–178.

O'Brien-Pallas, L., Duffield, C., & Alksnis, C. (2004). Who will be there to nurse? Retention of nurses nearing retirement. *Journal of Nursing Administration, 34*(6), 298–302.

Stone, P. W., Harrison, M. I., Feldman, P., Linzer, M., Peng, T., Roblin, D., . . . Williams, E. S. (2005). Organizational climate of staff working conditions and safety—an integrative model. *Advances in Patient Safety: From Research to Implementation, 2,* 467–481.

U.S. Census Bureau. (2006a). *Accuracy of the data.* Retrieved from http://www.census.gov/acs/www/Downloads/ACS/accuracy2006.pdf

U.S. Census Bureau. (2006b). *American Community Survey/Puerto Rico Community Survey 2006 subject definitions.* Retrieved from http://www.census.gov/acs/www/Downloads/2006/usedata/Subject_Definitions.pdf

Wray, J., Aspland, J., Gibson, H., Stimpson, A., & Watson, R. (2009). "A wealth of knowledge": A survey of the employment experiences of older nurses and midwives in the NHS. *International Journal of Nursing Studies, 46*(7), 977–985.

2
Why Are Nurses With Disabilities Leaving Nursing?

John, a 35-year-old registered nurse, worked on a busy medical surgical floor. He loved the work and enjoyed the fast pace and daily challenge. Quite suddenly, he suffered an injury that resulted in traumatic hearing loss in both ears. He had no other injuries. He grieved the loss but was eligible for hearing aids and learned to read lips. Hearing aids are expensive so he had to manage with only one hearing aid. His nurse manager acquired an assistive device that was placed on one of the phones at the nurses' station for his use. It took some adjustment, but he thought he was managing to care for his patients quite well. Initially, his colleagues and his supervisor were sympathetic and attentive. However, he soon found it difficult to use the phone because the assistive device was frequently detached from the phone by other people who didn't need to use it. He had a hard time locating it and sometimes had to give up. He also found himself frequently reminding staff to face him when they spoke to him but this was often forgotten. He was aware that patients and their families thought he was ignoring them. He taught himself to explain his disability to each of his patients and their families. After awhile, John found that he was not able to keep up his usual pace and efficiency because he couldn't make phone calls and he had to keep reminding staff to speak directly to him. He had asked his manager to give him written reports of all meetings so he could make sure he didn't miss anything important but this too fell by the wayside. When John would ask his manager to repeat things at meetings, everyone teased him about being hard of hearing. Finally, John decided to leave the job and he found a job in nursing informatics. He was able to use the computer in his work. He missed his previous nursing work terribly but was unsure of how to continue in bedside care despite the disability.

Nurses with disabilities are leaving nursing. The research (Guillett, Neal-Boylan, & Lathrop, 2007; Neal-Boylan & Guillett, 2008a, 2008b,

2008c) done thus far indicates that nurses with physical and/or sensory disabilities leave nursing for a variety of reasons. This chapter will address why nurses with disabilities are leaving nursing and offer suggestions regarding how the profession might retain them.

OVERVIEW

Nurses with disabilities often perceive that they are being pushed out of their jobs. Even nurses who have acknowledged expertise and longevity within a particular area of nursing perceive that others no longer accept them as fully capable to do their jobs because of the disability. This perception is manifested in a variety of ways. Sometimes nurses feel that others resent them when they do not have the stamina or energy to float to other units or work the evening or night shifts. Often, nurses with disabilities get the sense that others are resentful or skeptical when they cannot lift patients or perform certain physical tasks.

Sometimes, nurses with disabilities are made to feel isolated from their "well" colleagues such as the nurse whose office was given to someone else while she was a patient in the hospital and when she returned, her new office was far removed from the offices of her colleagues. Occasionally, the views of colleagues and administrators are verbally or physically expressed to the nurse but more often, the nurse simply realizes that her or his colleagues may not feel about them the way they had previously.

DIFFICULTY MEETING EXPECTATIONS

One nurse who had had a hip replacement found that walking long distances was difficult so she was told by her health care provider to work only on her unit because everything was accessible. Her personal physician gave her a note of support. The nurses on her unit thought that she was trying to avoid floating to other units or avoiding work. This perception, that the nurse is trying to get out of work, seems pervasive. Others seem threatened by the nurse's valid "excuses" to avoid certain kinds of work or to use compensatory techniques to enable them to accomplish their work.

A hospital floor nurse who has limited function in one of her legs, had surgery and then needed to temporarily use crutches when she returned to work. Initially she was assigned paperwork and was moved into doing desk work that was needed on the unit. The other nurses made it clear that she was receiving favoritism even though the paperwork was necessary and someone had to do it and it made perfect sense for her to be the one to do it while she recovered. The nurse was put in a very difficult position because she was doing much of her supervisor's work without receiving any recognition for it and was told that she had to "pretend" to be doing a floor nursing job.

> [I was told] that the hospital wasn't creating any new positions. . . . [They said] we're just gonna continue to pretend that this is what you're doing, you're filling your job description but you're just doing projects on the side as extra work.

In addition, she had to wait to get the tools she needed to do the new work such as a phone and a computer.

> It took me 9 months to get my own computer and I would be going back and forth. . . . One of the doctors that works in the unit graciously offered to let me put another desk in her office so that I could at least have a hub . . . to sit at to do the work that I was asked to do but I didn't get a computer until just a couple [of] months ago. . . . It's an attention drawer. If you need a computer and that's a lot of money, plus all the software that goes on the computer to make my job possible, plus then a phone where people can contact me and you're saying that you're gonna put an extension with my name on it, you know it draws attention so I understand why my boss wouldn't want to do that, but at the same time, those were the things I needed. . . . But once I did get a computer? Oh man, that started a riot. . . .

This nurse felt like things in her case could've been handled differently because if they had been, she might have made different choices.

> I would've liked to have been afforded the opportunity to look at [the options] instead of having it be that every day I'm on eggshells waiting almost a year and a half. . . . I wish that I had known that this could potentially happen—be told that I'm not fulfilling a job requirement so that I could make some choices or look outside of the hospital, focus full time on school, something. . . .

This nurse, like so many others with disabilities, was not offered options for how she could stay in nursing or within the organization despite the disability. She ended up going back to school for a degree outside of nursing. She also ended up switching jobs. ". . . I [just] got notified [that] a place that I interviewed [with] . . . is making an offer so I will be putting in my 2 weeks' notice and saying sayonara."

Nurse sometimes leave because they feel limited in what they can do by pain or reduced stamina and strength. At other times, they sense that they are being pushed out or are fired for some other reason that they feel largely had to do with their disability. One nurse found that she could only work at certain times of the day because of a neuromuscular condition.

> I found that my better times were in the morning and as the afternoon progressed my ability to do much of anything sort of decreased, preventing me from working overtime, preventing me from working late hours. Of course, this did not sit well with my co-workers who were then required to work the later hours so I could work the earlier hours.

This problem was reiterated by another nurse:

> ... They require you to float wherever else they want you to go and I can't do that right now. With my fibromyalgia, I've got to get so many hours of sleep or that adds up. So, I can't do night shifts.... There were nurses complaining that I couldn't do my job like other people. The other nurses have to float. The other nurses have to go to x-ray with their patient. The other nurses ... said that with me not floating and with me not going to nights and not going over with the patients on the x-ray on some weekends, I was not a team player.... So they, in turn, fired me.

BEING TREATED DIFFERENTLY

To add insult to injury, the nurse described above was targeted during a special meeting in which the director of the department asked all of the staff how they felt about this nurse being treated as "special" (the nurse's quotation marks).

> Oh, it was awful. It was like an inquisition.... I felt like crying. I just kept thinking these are my co-workers, these are people and also nurses and they are all sitting here looking at me like I'm somebody who asked to get this disease. I didn't ask to get [this disease]. Please, that was the furthest thing from my mind. I always figured [I'd] end up getting cancer because that is what is in the family.

This nurse was specifically told by Human Resources at the facility that a position would not be created for her nor were accommodations going to be made. "Well, you would think that working in a health care facility that they might have a little bit of empathy toward one of their own but no, all I got was animosity and people who thought I was getting special treatment." This summarizes an interesting finding that despite being health care professionals, neither nurses nor physicians tend to support each other when one of them has an illness or disability (Neal-Boylan, 2012; Neal-Boylan et al., 2012).

This nurse was initially shifted out of the operating room, which she had loved, and into the ambulatory surgery unit for admitting and discharging patients. However, when she could not work the later hours, she was not supported and further problems began. After this was when Human Resources declined to place her elsewhere within the organization. Chapter 6 discusses, in detail, the interactions nurses with disabilities have within the work environment and how these interactions impact their job termination.

DECIDING TO LEAVE

Nurses with disabilities often leave their jobs voluntarily. They may feel that they can no longer manage the tasks required of them; they may sense resentment from others and not want to work in a hostile environment that makes them feel uncomfortable and unappreciated for the knowledge and skills they have. Many nurses recognize that it is difficult for them, their patients, and other staff if they continue to work in a particular environment. In these cases, nurses with disabilities do not express their resentment of others for making them feel like they need to leave, but feel that they are doing their best by their patients and colleagues if they leave the position. However, when the nurse voluntarily leaves a position such as critical care because he or she cannot maneuver around or respond as quickly as is needed, they reasonably expect the facility and nurse administrators to help them relocate to another position within the facility or agency so they can remain with the organization and continue to work in nursing. According to the nurses studied, this rarely happens. Instead, the nurse is allowed, and often encouraged to leave, and does not receive assistance to find another position within the organization. How often this happens generally is not precisely known but that it does happen all too much is clear. At the same time, colleagues are sometimes supportive but administrators are not and they make the final decisions. As one nurse said: "I've really been in a very supportive environment. I really can't complain at all in terms of my coworkers. In terms of administration? That's another whole story." Consequently, there is a significant and unnecessary loss of nursing experience and expertise that might otherwise be retained and put to good use. One nurse said: "I just can't do nursing right now. I'm not well enough. . . . And I was born a nurse. I mean, I'm one of these people who always knew I was gonna be a nurse."

REPERCUSSIONS

Interestingly, relatively few nurses seem to file any legal claims of discrimination or request disability compensation. This was also true of physicians with disabilities who were interviewed (Neal-Boylan, 2012; Neal-Boylan et al., 2012). In the cases of the nurses, they appeared reluctant to cause any trouble or to admit that they weren't wanted or couldn't stay in the current position. A glaring case involved a nurse with physical disabilities who was offered a position to develop a new program but felt that her acquiescence to a romantic relationship with the supervisor was pivotal to retaining the job. She left and chose not to report the sexual harassment.

> It was awful. I guess I needed to leave anyway, but I knew that I couldn't work on the floor. I finished what I had to do and . . . thought, I can't stay here. I'm not gonna offend the head of nursing but I'm not gonna go out with her either.

Nurse are often not aware of the laws or their rights with regard to disability and it appears that they are rarely, if ever, informed about their options unless they press the issue. A nurse with rheumatoid arthritis filed for medical leave after a family member told her she had the right to do so. Human Resources and management in the hospital where she worked did not give her this information until she approached them. She filed for medical leave but did not know she had to renew this yearly.

> [Human Resources] didn't notify me that after a year I had to refile the paperwork so as soon as my one year was up . . . they tried to come after me again. I had to get involved with human resources and get the paperwork in and then I was aware of it so the next year then I made sure that I got that signed and then that was the year they reworked my position. . . . I feel like [they] definitely [wanted] to get me out of there and [they did not] understand that some of the things that they were seeing were issues. I truly feel like if at any point they would've sat down with me and just said these are the things that we're seeing as a problem it would have helped me to look . . . at disability because I'm not fulfilling the expectations of the job, rather than just looking for a way to move me out of there.

This nurse was not provided with the information she needed to make informed choices.

> ... I felt like there was some resistance.... I did a lot of self-educating between my sister and resources she gave me before I even presented it to HR and I again felt like there was some resistance there ... not notifying me that their expectation was that I renew [FMLA] every year and my sister was pretty mortified, horrified by the fact that they were not more aware of what they needed to do in that situation and that I met that kind of resistance. I really felt like ... they complied only because once they knew I was educating myself and that I knew what the rules were and what their legal responsibilities were, they didn't have [a] choice but to comply. I think had I not done that I would've lost that job much earlier than I did.

The sense is that if the nurses don't ask then no one should tell them what their options are, whether the options pertain to other jobs within the organization or to their rights as individuals with disabilities.

Sometimes nurses are told by their physicians that they should stop nursing. One nurse with a neuromuscular disease had worked for 10 years before leaving nursing voluntarily. By this time she was having trouble standing. However, she eventually decided to try to go back to work "because they needed my help but they don't seem to be able to find a way to let me help. They didn't say as much but I could see that they need help. ... I think they would rather have someone that could walk; they prefer ambulation."

When this nurse was asked if anything could facilitate her return to work, she answered "There is not, because they have people that are afraid and they don't listen to me, they have a lot of fear." When asked what they, meaning administrators, are afraid of, she said "ME. taking their jobs or if I have a niche for myself and I would be taking away their opportunities." This nurse was not informed of other nursing opportunities within the organization. "It was suggested that I should retire. I think maybe they didn't know what I could do."

CONCERN FOR PATIENT SAFETY

Sometimes nurses with disabilities leave because they fear they will jeopardize patient safety. It is interesting to note that to date, there has been no published record of a nurse jeopardizing patient safety because of a physical and/or sensory disability. In a study of nurses and physicians with disabilities, it was interesting to find that both groups worried about jeopardizing patient safety and took great pains to avoid any possible harm to the patient (Neal-Boylan, 2012; Neal-Boylan et al., 2012). (Chapter 5 addresses this issue in detail.) However, nurses put patients first. Nurses with disabilities often say that they do not want to do anything that might possibly hurt the patient either because the nurse missed something, such as in the case of a hearing impairment, or because the nurse could not perform a procedure or intervention safely. One nurse said: "I think there's some accommodations they can make, but you can only go so far. If my hearing were really bad in this ear, I probably wouldn't be able to do it. . . . It'd be really hard, period."

One nurse left nursing because of an acute onset of traumatic hearing loss. She was not deaf but had hearing impairment and obtained hearing aids. Despite the hearing aids, she did not go back to work. She described being afraid to go back because she might not hear her patients. After the hearing loss, she briefly went back to work before she realized how severe the hearing loss was.

> I knew that when they gave report I'd say "what was that . . . what did you [say?]" and they'd look at me like "what do you want to do read my lips?" And I realized it slightly but . . . it's just denial. And I couldn't accept that, I couldn't just fit back in.

WHO IS LEAVING?

Nurses with chronic diseases or who have had injuries that affect their mobility or dexterity and nurses who have some or severe difficulty communicating, hearing or seeing appear to be leaving nursing (Neal-Boylan, Fennie, & Baldauf-Wagner, 2011). Nurses who have to in some way change their schedules (due to the need to eat at certain times or due to fatigue and energy limitations) or do things differently from the traditional, accepted ways of doing things are also leaving nursing. Nurses who appear to be very willing and able to use reasonable accommodations to be able to function effectively as nurses are leaving their jobs, often because no one offers or is willing to provide those accommodations. Nurses who need to sit instead of stand for prolonged periods or walk frequently or for long distances are also leaving. Nurses who cannot perform in settings where they were able to work prior to the onset of disability often leave voluntarily or they may be pushed out, but they are rarely offered options so they can stay within the organization.

As this book will discuss, sometimes nurses leave because they feel they cannot do the work and sometimes they are encouraged—whether subtly or not—to leave. Sometimes it is appropriate for nurses to leave their current setting so that others who can meet the physical demands can take their places for the benefit of the patient. However, these nurses are not assisted to find other work in nursing, either from their own organizations or from national nursing organizations who might be in a position to provide guidance or assistance.

There does not seem to be an overall willingness to try to accommodate jobs so that the organization can retain the nurse's expertise. Nurses shifts are not decreased or their work load reduced. Very little support is provided to help them use the phone if they have problems hearing or to move and lift patients by encouraging other staff to help the colleague with a disability. There seems to be a general expectation that the nurse will either do the whole job the way it was intended or not do the job at all, with little thought given to whether small changes could be made to retain the nurse.

Chapter 1 of this book discussed the types of disabilities encountered during the studies of nurses with disabilities. These disabilities ranged from severe allergies to mobility and musculoskeletal problems, neurological impairments, and chronic diseases and included both congenital and acquired disabilities. Most of these nurses had either left a nursing position because of reasons related to the disability or had left the profession altogether. Clearly, the problem of retaining nurses with disabilities is one that is significant to nursing. Particularly as nurses age and people of all walks of life continue to live with chronic illnesses and disabilities, the likelihood of there being more nurses with disabilities of some kind than there are now will increase. It behooves the nursing profession to find ways of keeping these nurses in the profession. It is also vital that nursing recognize that if it discourages potential nursing students with disabilities from entering nursing programs, it stands to lose a substantial number of highly qualified, intelligent people to the profession.

Nurses with disabilities experience a wide variety of symptoms. Sometimes they have had these symptoms for a long period of time and might even come to the job with them. At other times, they develop symptoms acutely and find themselves suddenly having to integrate symptom management into their personal and professional lives. One nurse explained:

> ... Literally one day waking up and not being able to flex my fingers that were all tingling. Prior to that, I had had an unusual amount of fatigue. I had weight loss, significant weight loss.

I had been feeling really ill when I woke up in the morning with pounding, pounding headaches, which I never [used to] get. And also I had some episodes with tendonitis and some issues with my shoulder and spine. And in retrospect . . . I realized that a lot of those things can be precursors to an acute onset or to a diagnosis.

Another nurse described a sudden onset of symptoms.

I started to have leg pain, sharp stabbing pains down my leg. It proceeded to get worse and I kept working and then . . . my back started to hurt, my lower back. . . . The pain was all the time, so I was unable to really do anything at my job. I would always have pain if I needed to bend over and do a dressing change or pick something up, if I needed to do anything at all really.

Another nurse found herself with paralysis of her lower extremities and wheelchair-bound. ". . . Once I was told that I was permanently disabled, I just couldn't accept that." This nurse was a supervisor in a psychiatric unit at the time of the onset of her paralysis. At the time she was interviewed, she was in negotiation to get her job back. At that point she could walk about 400 feet with a lot of assistance.

This nurse described feeling supported by her colleagues who visited her but she felt that more could have been done by the facility to facilitate her return to work and to make accommodations for her. "I have this label. . . . It's hard to keep fighting." The nurse hired an attorney. "I have tried to handle this on my own, but it's so overwhelming." The nurse described feeling angry and saying that she had distanced herself from her previous employers because of the hassle and frustration. She described being told that she was an excellent employee on initial review and that she had had great annual reviews ever since. There had never been any complaints against her. Despite this, it appeared to her at the time of the research interview that the organization was not willing to make accommodations and still expected her to work 12 hour shifts. She did not see why a return to work would be a problem as her job had primarily consisted of "solving problems. I can still solve problems."

Others have had symptoms for a long period of time but they become less manageable or less difficult to hide or compensate for at work. "I have uneven strength in my arms. I have fatigue that's overwhelming. I have braces on my legs and my hands and the fatigue, the absolute fatigue is the hardest thing for me." Another nurse encountered problems with her allergies despite hospital rules regarding perfumes and smoking.

[I am] allergic to cigarette smoke and perfumes but [the hospital] had a rule where you [weren't] supposed to wear scented stuff to

> work or anything like that, but they still had it so some patients could smoke in the hospital and staff could smoke in the break room. But the break room was where you gave report. . . . So, I got completely disabled because of my breathing. [When] they came out with the smoking thing and you were not able to smoke in the hospitals anymore, that kind of helped . . . to a point but at the same time, all the people that were smoking go outside the front door and smoke so when you come to work you had to go through them to get into the building and that would set my asthma off.

The nurse described moving to a different hospital in which colleagues were understanding about her allergies and didn't wear perfume. However, the cleaning products used caused her breathing difficulties. The facility accommodated her by having the cleaning done after she finished her shift and left the hospital.

Later, this nurse decided to become a traveling nurse but encountered less hospitable environments and people less willing to accommodate her. At one point, she told an administrator: "When you hired me, in your policy, it says no scented lotions, deodorants, perfumes . . . [there's] all these people wearing it. I have to report it because I can't breathe." When the nurse was told that others had as much right to wear their perfume and scents as she had, she contacted the Disabilities Rights Commission and they provided some help. "But nobody seemed to care . . . and the other nurses gave me more static on it than [the] patients [did]." In many cases, this nurse found that patients and families, once informed that the unit preferred that perfumes and scents be kept to a minimum, were more likely to comply than the staff.

Symptoms do not only affect nurses in physically demanding jobs. Academic nurses and researchers also experience difficulties related to their symptoms. Fatigue is a common symptom among nurses with disabilities that often affects the work nurses do.

> The last job I had was doing research but I would fall asleep in meetings. I was unable to learn the new studies that we had gotten and also . . . I was putting in data for somebody and they told me it was all wrong. . . . I got raked over the coals for falling asleep in a meeting. [I] was told "well if you're gonna fall asleep and you're tired, then you shouldn't come to work." And I tried to explain "I don't know when I'm gonna get tired."

This nurse got an attorney's help to get her an accommodation so she didn't have to work at night because she had been taking night call as part of a research project. "I needed accommodation that I couldn't do night calls and they gave me a hard time, [saying that] it was an essential part of the job.... They were anything but understanding." Later, this nurse began to have problems with her balance and had some falls. After one fall, "my colleagues saw me and immediately ran and told my supervisor."

> And that did it.... She said "We need to talk" and she took me into HR [Human Resources] after this meeting. We went back to my office. [I] tried to get into my computer and could not. [I] went to HR and was basically told "Since you have short-term and long-term disability [insurance], you ought to take advantage of it." And I said, "Well, okay." And they said "and you can go ahead and leave now." ... I didn't get to talk to anybody.

At the time of the research interview, the nurse said that there had been no further contact "to try to get me back or part time or anything. It was just—they basically kicked me out the door."

Not all of the disabilities nurses have are severe or severely limiting. The reader should not get the impression that only nurses with severe illnesses or disabilities are being pushed out of nursing and then in some way feel that this is justified. Most nurses interviewed felt that there was something they could do that would employ their expertise even if they had a disability and most of the nurses were still made to feel unwanted at work even if their disability was mild or moderate.

Sensory impairments also often result in disability for nurses and influence their work lives. Some, such as nurses who have trouble hearing, use augmented equipment. Sometimes equipment they place on the telephones at work so they can take and make phone calls is inadvertently removed by others. It can be hard for nurses with hearing disabilities to work in some settings.

> Sometimes, [people] may be behind you and talking. You don't even know they're talking to you. And I've heard visitors make comments: "Well he's not even paying attention." I say "Well, I'm sorry. I didn't know you were talking to me."

One study found that nurses with trouble hearing were more likely to leave hospital work than to leave other nursing settings (Neal-Boylan et al., 2011).

Often a sense of humor helps the nurse with a disability to cope. An ability to laugh at oneself can soften words that are said by others out of ignorance or insensitivity. One nurse with a hearing impairment used humor to make his colleagues feel more at ease with his disability but also to remind them of his need for occasional assistance.

Sometimes, instead of using the intercom system from the nurses' station, they'll (the nurses) yell something and I can't hear them. Then they say, "I can't hear you." I say "well, I can only hear out of one ear. How am I supposed to hear you when you can't even hear me and you got two good ears?"

EMOTIONS

Sometimes the nurse discovers that the job she or he took on is really much more than they can manage and there are subsequent feelings of frustration and grief associated with the decision to leave the job.

> I started out full time and I couldn't do it. I just couldn't do it. The job was so much more than what I could manage . . . I could work 3 days. I just couldn't do a whole day, and I think after that job, I really gave up. I gave up hoping that I could do anything and then I went into a period of real depression over all these changes 'cause I felt that I had done a lot of adjusting. I worked a lot of different places and still had something to give but I did not know how to give it. . . .

Another nurse described her reaction when she found out that she had suffered traumatic hearing loss and felt that she could not longer work safely as a nurse: "It was very traumatic. And then I didn't realize how much I had lost until people kept bringing it up to me, that . . . [the] television set is so loud . . . you're rattling the windows."

Often, the need to leave nursing seems unfair and unnecessary. This is why so many nurses with disabilities perceive that they are targets of discrimination. One nurse said:

> I always loved nursing. I loved what I did and I miss it so much but I tell you what really, really irritated me was when one of the nurses was caught with a substance that was illegal, she was counseled and when she came back she was given light duty. She was given a duty telephoning patients and making assessments, that kind of thing and I said "you know what?" I could have done that job. Why wasn't that job offered to me?

Another nurse said, regarding having a disability, that you begin to question yourself and whether or not you should remain in nursing.

> Should I be here? Should I be doing this? Maybe I shouldn't be doing this. . . . You start questioning yourself and thinking "Do

they like that? Do they [not] like that? Am I right? Am I wrong? Who's doing this? Who's doing that?" It really gets to be so much stress. It's always in the back of my mind. . . . I worry about what other people are thinking.

A nurse with rheumatoid arthritis explained:

. . . basically what you learn when you go though this is everybody pretty much is all for themselves. They're not concerned about anyone else. . . . I couldn't wait till summer [to have surgery] it was just too severe so as soon as I knew I had a scheduled time for the surgery, I called my supervisor and her response was "Well I have to see what I can do to save your job." That was her response. So, I knew I had to go through with what I had to go through with. I had no choice. . . . Within a week of having surgery, they sent me a letter. . . . They wanted me to go to a termination hearing. . . . Nobody said anything about that till after the fact and I did let my supervisor know [that] if anything else had to be done, I would have done it but I didn't know. I think I was being set up in a way. I think it was their opportunity to get rid of me because of the physical problems.

This nurse was terminated and in her view the reason was that she had knee surgery. She found another job and hid her disability at the interview but when her manager realized that she couldn't run or easily negotiate steps, she found that the manager did not support her.

Inwardly you are [on the defensive]. I will have to say because of that, maybe my perceptions as a result of my very bad experience—because it was devastating to me—maybe it skewed my perception of things after that when I have been in the work place. Maybe I was overly sensitive. Maybe I read too much into things. I don't know but I think it's possible. I do know that for that job I was doing a good job. The nurse that was training me said I was doing wonderful[ly] and I didn't have a problem with her. It was just this nurse manager. She could see that I couldn't run like the rest of them. They could run.

Another nurse spoke of having to leave her hospital job because of her disability but that she eventually found nursing work that she could do within the limits of her disability. While she was out of nursing temporarily, she grieved for the loss of her nursing identity.

. . . It was real hard to move out of clinical nursing into a different type of role. . . . Honestly, the biggest identity crisis I've ever gone through was the three years I wasn't working at all and my nursing license lapsed because I found all of a sudden I didn't know how to introduce myself to people because I'd always been: "I'm X, I'm a nurse." All of a sudden it was like, "I'm X, I'm a nurse. I *was* a nurse." It was like I didn't realize how much being a nurse had become a part of my identity. . . . There was a little bit of that in making the transition but it was much harder when I was not working at all and didn't have my license because— okay, what am I? [Now I can say]. . . . Yes, I am a nurse, I don't work clinically but I am a nurse.

HOW DO WE KEEP THEM FROM LEAVING?

Many nurses with disabilities have vast expertise in nursing that the profession cannot afford to lose. It is striking how many nurses with disabilities say that no one assisted them to stay in their organizations in a different position or bothered to discuss potential accommodations that could be made so they could continue their jobs. One nurse recruiter said:

> There are times when you know the person in front of you cannot possibly do the work, they cannot meet the requirements of the job description and there is no point in wasting the individual's time or the organization's time and money by continuing the process. I'll give you an example. . . . A person came in for an interview and when she arrived, she was very short of breath and puffing, sort of sounded asthmatic and even worse, actually looked a little gray. It is a long walk in from the parking lot and into the buildings so, of course, it was offered that she sit for a minute and catch her breath, etc., before beginning and she volunteered that oh, this was her usual state. Well, there is no way that she would have been able to pass the physical, even so there was no point in sending her forward. . . . This woman could not even make it down the hallway without being compromised, let alone carry out the expectations of the job.

Might it have been possible to consider this nurse for a job in which walking down hallways was not necessary? Were her skills, experience, and expertise considered or was she dismissed out of hand? It is worth wondering how many nurse recruiters and managers had turned this nurse away and whether anyone had considered offering her something that would retain her in nursing and make use of her abilities within the organization. According to the law, if she was eligible for the job in ways unrelated to her disability, she should've been offered the job, given the medical examination, and then she could have legitimately been told that she could not meet the physical demands of the job. Instead it appears that the decision regarding whether or not to hire her was based on her disability.

Staying within the organization might be affected by the nurse's tolerance for pain and stigma, but often they have little control over whether or not they can stay. Sometimes a nurse, knowing he or she has a particular disability, seeks out a certain type of nursing job that the nurse feels he or she can do and of which others will be supportive. (Chapter 4 discusses how having a disability affects the job and career choices of the nurse with a disability.) One nurse described applying for a job in college health because she knew what her capabilities were and what the job would entail.

> I'd done college nursing for quite some time before I had the diagnosis.... So, I kind of knew what the job required and it's not like bedside medical surgical ICU (intensive care unit) nursing.... I knew I'd be able to handle it quite well but I don't know [that] they really talked to me anything specific about it.

This nurse was able to compensate for certain things in her job and there were also things that she didn't have to do to fulfill her role.

> ... You learn how to position yourself differently if something's uncomfortable but basically a lot of what I do is like an outpatient clinic versus an inpatient setting. I don't have to lift patients. I don't have to turn patients. I don't have to do a lot of physical stuff with my job which if I were in ... a hospital situation, I don't think I'd still be in nursing at this point. I'm almost positive I would not be.

Nurses with disabilities leave nursing because, while they typically recognize that they cannot, nor would they consider themselves capable of doing every type of job in nursing, they do not know what jobs are yet open to them. This is partly due to stories like the one above in which a judgment was made about the nurse, probably before she could discuss her abilities, and partly because no one makes an effort to assist the nurse to find a job he or she can do. Nurses themselves must be willing to investigate what is possible and many do, but others become so discouraged by how they are treated or ignored that they become disillusioned with the profession itself.

What Can Nurse Educators Do?

Nurse educators can integrate discussions about nurses and other health care professionals with disabilities into lessons regarding chronic illness and the care of the patient with a disability. Instilling a sense of camaraderie for all fellow nurses and colleagues, including those with disabilities, might go a long way to restoring the esprit de corps that once characterized nursing. Dispelling this notion (discussed further in Chapter 3) that nurses must heroically and bravely forge ahead despite pain, fatigue, and disability and without making any compensations or changes in the *way* they do their jobs would potentially help all nurses to feel that they are allowed to be human and can rely on their colleagues for physical and emotional support when times are hard. Nurse educators should be teaching students about rehabilitation theory and the resources available to people with disabilities anyway, so it is reasonable that they should expand this discussion to include nurses and health care colleagues in the workplace in this discussion.

Nurse academe should make schools of nursing welcoming to people with physical and/or sensory disabilities by valuing prospective students for the intelligence they bring to nursing. Ways of changing how we educate nursing students to accommodate people with disabilities are discussed in detail in Chapter 8.

What Can Nurse Leaders Do?

Nurse leaders should set the example by encouraging nurses both within and outside of the clinical setting to demonstrate esprit de corps to one another and to practice what they preach by modeling for patients and families how people with disabilities and chronic illnesses should be treated: with respect and an emphasis on abilities rather than on disabilities. Nursing is replete with professional organizations that have myriad opportunities to educate and inform their members about how we can better care for one another. Further, nursing organizations should offer electronic databases and other technology that could utilize a nurse's demographic information and information regarding their *abilities* and direct them to job opportunities that might be able to accommodate them if they have a disability. Nurses with disabilities with expertise in informatics could develop this technology and administer it, as only nurses truly know what nurses are looking for in their jobs.

There needs to be an increased awareness that nurses with disabilities are leaving the profession and that we cannot afford to lose them. Nurses have always been creative thinkers. Recognition will surely lead to new ideas regarding how to better incorporate nurses with disabilities into the work of nursing so they don't leave nursing, for any reason.

REFERENCES

Guillett, S. E., Neal-Boylan, L. J., & Lathrop, R. (2007). Ready, willing, and disabled. *American Nurse Today, 2*(8), 30–32.

Neal-Boylan, L. J. (2012). An exploration and comparison of the worklife experiences of registered nurses and physicians with permanent physical and/or sensory disabilities. *Rehabilitation Nursing, 37*(1), 3–10.

Neal-Boylan, L. J., Fennie, K., & Baldauf-Wagner, S. (2011). Nurses with sensory disabilities: Their perceptions and characteristics. *Rehabilitation Nursing, 36*(1), 25–31.

Neal-Boylan, L. J., & Guillett, S. E. (2008a). Nurses with disabilities: Can changing our educational system keep them in nursing? *Nurse Educator, 33*(4), 1–4.

Neal-Boylan, L. J., & Guillett, S. E. (2008b). Registered nurses with physical disabilities. *Journal of Nursing Administration, 38*(1), 1–3.

Neal-Boylan, L. J., & Guillett, S. E. (2008c). Work experiences of RNs with physical disabilities. *Rehabilitation Nursing, 33*(2), 67–72.

Neal-Boylan, L. J., Hopkins, A., Skeete, R., Hartmann, S. B., Iezzoni, L. I., & Nunez-Smith, M. (2012). The career trajectories of health care professionals practicing with permanent disabilities. *Academic Medicine, 87*(2), 172–178.

3
Hiding the Disability

Martha, a 42-year-old RN with fibromyalgia and diabetes mellitus type 2, applied for a job at a large urban hospital on their medical floor. Martha has frequent fatigue and widespread muscle tenderness throughout her body. She also takes medication for her diabetes and must eat at regular intervals to avoid hypoglycemic episodes. She is an experienced nurse and has just moved to a new state. Martha receives a phone call asking her to appear for an interview. The interview goes well and the nurse recruiter is very impressed with Martha's résumé and experience. Martha does not disclose that she has two chronic illnesses and how they affect her. She is hired for the job, fills out the necessary paperwork and is told she will have a complete physical exam by a nurse practitioner on the hospital staff. If all goes well, Martha will begin work in 2 weeks. She is very excited and calls her husband to tell him the news. During the physical exam, Martha reveals to the nurse practitioner that she has fibromyalgia and diabetes and lists her medications. She says that as long as she is able to take the breaks allotted by the job (lunch and two 15-minute breaks during the shift) and can eat on schedule, she should be fine. The nurse practitioner passes her and Martha begins work 2 weeks later. Martha's medical floor is very busy and consequently, the nurses hardly ever get their breaks and often catch meals when they can while charting. To her surprise, Martha is placed on the evening shift and is unable to get home before midnight. She wakes early to get her children off to school. When Martha meets with her manager and explains that the inability to eat at regular times and to get her necessary rest are impeding her ability to function at her best, her manager states that Martha's illnesses and disabilities were not brought up when she was initially hired and that she cannot do anything to ameliorate Martha's concerns because she doesn't want to be unfair to the other nurses. Eventually, Martha has to leave this job because she is unable to reach an agreement with her manager. She is able to get an interview at a smaller community hospital in the area. Martha initially has a phone interview that is very positive and the recruiter asks her to come in for an in-person interview. This time,

> Martha reveals her medical history and her special needs to the nurse recruiter. Following this revelation, Martha notes that the recruiter's demeanor changes from welcoming and enthusiastic to more reserved. They finish the interview and the recruiter thanks her for coming. Martha never hears back about the job.

It is interesting to note that, when asked, many nurse recruiters—that is, a nurse who is often a nurse manager in the position of interviewing and hiring a nurse for a job—could not recall ever interviewing a nurse with a disability. This may be due to the tendency of nurses with disabilities who can hide their disabilities to do so and it may be due to reluctance by these nurse recruiters to admit that they had ever interviewed nurses with disabilities. The first part of this chapter will discuss the perceptions of nurse recruiters and managers regarding the hiring practices of nurses with disabilities. The next section will present the perceptions of nurses with disabilities regarding hiding the disabilities. Finally, potential solutions to this problem will be discussed.

NURSE RECRUITERS AND MANAGERS

According to the law, one cannot ask about the disability or the extent of the disability during the hiring process, but one can ask whether the person can do the job. Interestingly, when asked, many nurse recruiters do not remember interviewing or hiring a nurse with an obvious disability. This is consistent with the finding that many nurses with disabilities hide their disabilities from recruiters and managers.

Nurse recruiters and managers were hard to recruit for research participation because they expressed concern about their employers and others finding out about what they had to say. Repeated assurances of anonymity eventually won the day in most of these cases. However, it raises a red flag that recruiters and managers might be reluctant to speak about what happens in their facilities. It indicates that they realize that situations involving nurses with disabilities may not always be handled in a lawful or ethical way but they may feel pressured to do what they are told.

> It's kind of interesting because most people come in for interviews and you don't really see whether they have a disability or not and we are not allowed to ask about disabilities and unless the person you're speaking with mentions it to you, there really isn't a way unless it's obvious that they have a physical problem.

REQUIREMENTS TO WORK

When asked if there are conditions that would affect a nurse's ability to practice, a variety were mentioned. One nurse recruiter cited the ability to "hear well" as necessary for functioning in critical care: ". . . you're expected to answer your own alarms, and those alarms have different rings. . . . So, I think . . . in critical care . . . that would be pretty essential."

Is the ability to hear essential to nursing practice? Anecdotally, and in the research, nurses with difficulty hearing often stated that if people made sure to look directly at them when they spoke, there was no difficulty understanding what the person was trying to communicate to them. Nurses with hearing problems also mention obtaining a device, whether from the facility or on their own, to attach to the phone to enable them to understand people on the phone. These nurses said that frequently the device was removed, inadvertently, by others and they could not locate the device when they needed to use the phone.

A nursing director in an academic setting commented on the nurse's ability to speak:

> Probably if they couldn't speak, it would be difficult to hire someone although we could probably make some kind of arrangement but I think it would be difficult if it was a problem with someone's voice because this job has a lot to do with being able to present and speak out loud. . . . I think for the most part we can accommodate mobility problems. There are particular jobs where a mobility problem would be an issue. For example, if someone worked in the labs where they had to show students physically how to lift a patient and they were unable to do that, we would then have to have someone in the lab that could actually do the skill while the person with the disability was directing it. That would be a little expensive for me but it still could be done.

One nurse with a disability verified this perception that faculty had to be able to lift. It would seem reasonable that the educator could describe the lift and coach the students to perform it. Students could also watch a video or DVD that would show how to lift a patient and then the instructor could walk students through the mechanics of it without actually having to lift the person or a manikin. In the academic setting, there is an ever increasing use of simulation manikins and models to demonstrate what nurses previously showed students how to do on a live patient. These simulation models could be used for a variety of things that would enable an educator with disabilities to continue to teach.

If it is possible in an academic setting to have someone else do the lifting or complete the physical task that cannot be easily done by the nurse with a disability, then why is it difficult to envision doing the same in a facility or institution? In an academic setting, the nurse is instructing others how to perform a skill. In a clinical setting, the nurse can and should do this as well and could therefore be valued for what he or she brings to the organization by virtue of higher education and critical thinking.

Another nurse manager described certain skills within her setting that the nurse would have to be able to perform to work there.

> In my setting, there really might be a few disabilities that wouldn't adapt well and whether we could make up for that with technology is [questionable]. There [are] keyboarding skills. If somebody weren't able to use their hands, would we as a department be able to afford the adaptable equipment to get them set so that they could still perform the job? That would be the question. . . . As long as you can answer the phone. Somebody that wasn't able to speak obviously would not do the job. . . . A lot of nursing is physical and sometimes, I think it is a little tough to find out what's out there. Just because not enough information is out there, as far as what the options are.

The issue of whether or not the nurse has options goes to the heart of the need to hide the disability whenever possible. Nurses with physical disabilities appear to have few options to remaining in nursing. It is not that there are not jobs that are willing to accommodate the nurse or that there are not jobs that can be done despite the disability. Rather, it is a case, it appears, of a lack of awareness on the part of the nurse with a disability regarding the options and a lack of awareness and possibly willingness on the part of administrators to identify options so the nurse can remain within the organization.

Some nurse managers and recruiters described stringent physical requirements that could prevent a nurse with disabilities from being employed in a particular area. One manager described work on a psychiatric unit.

> We've had some folks that are unable to . . . stand for more than 35 or 45 minutes at a time. They would be required to do that while doing a group presentation. . . . We've tried to select them and place them in the work environment so that there are other people that can pick up those skills for them. But, once again, they need to pass a screening to be able to do certain things without exception, such as: They have to be able to lift 50 pounds, they need to be able

to be computer literate, being able to sit at the computer station at least for 30 minutes at a time, things of this nature.

Cardiopulmonary resuscitation (CPR) is another requirement of many nursing jobs. Some nurses with physical disabilities do not have the stamina or strength to do or continue CPR. The manager from the psychiatric unit was also concerned about a nurse who could not intervene safely with a patient who got out of control.

You would have to be able to guide a patient using firm direction. The mechanics involved are applying soft and hard restraints, being able to sit in an area for up to an hour and performing constant observations of the patient, suicide intervention, things of this nature.

This manager admitted that psychiatric nursing does present barriers to nurses with physical disabilities.

Sometimes, I think we are a little more cautious than other disciplines because we know how physical[ly] demanding being a psychiatric nurse can be. Especially on the inpatient unit today with the closure of state hospital beds, the acuity of our patients [is] much higher. We sometimes have folks that might be on a forensic unit. . . . We're a little more cautious and we're trying to be cognizant of the fact that we don't want to put that nurse in a situation where she or he could get additionally injured on top of having a physical disability.

When asked if there were conditions that would affect the ability of a nurse to work on that particular unit, the manager answered,

I think that you would have to take a look at the job description. . . . I think most job descriptions speak to the physical, what is required of people physically. So, there could be something that would be clearly outlined in the job description that may lead somebody to not qualify for the job based on job descriptions and the job requirements.

This nurse had difficulty defining disability and asked the interviewer to be specific. It was not uncommon during the interviews for nurse recruiters and nurse managers to be evasive when answering questions about nurses with disabilities and many people who said they would like to participate in the study declined because they suspected that their hiring practices were discriminatory according to the Americans with Disabilities Act (ADA). Even some of the recruiters who allowed themselves to be interviewed expressed concern that they might get into trouble if anyone found out they were describing their organization's hiring practices.

The issue of job description is an interesting one. In a recent study of nurses with disabilities (yet to be published), it was found that nurses frequently were not given job descriptions or that the job descriptions they were given were mere formalities and didn't match the actual work of the job. Sometimes, entirely different expectations were required than were delineated in the job description. In any case, none of the employed nurses with disabilities interviewed were unable to perform the tasks required in their job descriptions.

The job description appears to be a barrier and a mechanism by which recruiters and managers can effectively avoid hiring nurses with disabilities. A common thread among many nurse job descriptions continues to be the need to be able to lift a certain amount of weight.

> ... In order to pass your employee physical, you need to demonstrate with a physical therapist that you're able to lift over x number of pounds, that you're able to move a patient from a chair ergonomically correct for both you and for the patient. So, that's a condition of being hired, whether or not you pass your pre-employment physical which speaks to all of that.

Another nurse manager confirmed that if the nurse passed the physical exam requirement from the facility or agency "I would never know that the clinician has a disability, physical or emotional disabilities." This manager worked for a home care agency and confirmed that the lifting requirement was also true for home care.

The issue of having to lift patients is an interesting one. In a time when the profession strives to be recognized for its science and contributions to research, it is of some concern that lifting and physical labor continue to be integral parts of many job descriptions. In many cases, nurse's aides do the actual physical work of caring for the patient and the registered nurse is expected to design the plan of care and use his or her critical thinking skills to make changes in the plan and to respond quickly to changes in the patient's condition. Regarding the requirement to be able to lift, one nurse with a disability stated: "They're really compartmentalizing an entire group of people that can't meet the criteria and consequently can't fill the job." A nurse manager commented:

> I believe it [is] 50 pounds, you have to lift a big old square box and I had a hard time lifting it myself 'cause it's like a wooden box, it's

not like lifting a person. . . . You can be honest saying, well I hurt myself in the past . . . and that the doctor has a prescription saying how many pounds this clinician could lift so we know ahead of time. And if a clinician can only lift 20 pounds or 10 pounds, we have to accommodate those.

However when this manager was asked if anyone at the agency had ever been hired who was unable to lift the required amount, she responded that in 2 years, so she had not encountered anyone.

One nurse manager had an interesting perspective on the requirement of nurses to lift patients:

Nurses get hurt because nursing is the only profession in the world that thinks 100 pounds is light. You know if you go to [a factory] and you say to some big, rugged huge guy, pick up that box and move it over there which just weighs 100 pounds, he'll tell you to go pound sand, "that weighs 100 pounds! I'm not lifting that." But this itty bitty nurse will say, "Oh you know, Tilly only weighs 100 pounds. I'll transfer her and do her care by myself." It's just an odd phenomenon.

Another nurse manager in an office practice echoed the necessity to look at each job individually instead of standardizing the job requirements.

Well, it would depend on the job . . . and the requirements for the job. If the nurse is a staff nurse and needs to be able to manipulate patients or empty Foley catheters and she's chair bound, there would be certain things she could do and certain things she couldn't do so obviously that would have to be looked at. And then the individual with a disability would know the extent of her abilities and she would interview appropriately.

This implies that the nurse with disabilities is likely to reveal her or his disability but so many are reluctant or learn not to do so if at all possible, because the attitudes of recruiters and managers change once they spot a disability. This manager stated that she specifically looked for a place to work that was accommodating to people with disabilities. She acknowledged that the work of an RN in an office practice is less stringent than the expectations of a nurse in another type of setting. "I think an office position like this might be an ideal situation for a nurse with a disability."

Should nurses be valued for what they bring to their jobs by way of their knowledge, expertise, and ability to provide care and comfort? When asked what positive things nurses with disabilities bring to the clinical environment, one nurse manager said:

> They bring whatever they've got in the first place. Either they have positive things or they didn't, whether they have a disability, I think would be irrelevant. When you come into the climate, you bring warmth and goodness to the climate or you bring chill into the climate and whether or not you have a disability probably doesn't really matter much unless the disability brought you more humanity and now you're more human.

HIDDEN FROM RECRUITERS

Often nurses with disabilities who are able to conceal their disabilities will do so because they fear not being hired or being at a disadvantage. In fact, most of the nurse recruiters and managers interviewed could not recall ever knowingly hiring anyone with a physical disability. One nurse manager said:

> I'm trying to think. I've hired many nurses over the years ... there's nothing that immediately comes to mind as far as an obvious disability, like, perhaps they were in a wheelchair or unable to ambulate. So, for now, I'd have to say I'm not aware of anyone I've hired with a physical disability that we've perhaps talked about at the time of hiring.

The issue of the hidden disability is prevalent among nurses and physicians with disabilities (Neal-Boylan, 2012; Neal-Boylan et al., 2012). When asked whether she had ever hired a nurse with a physical disability, one nurse manager said no and then said she was not sure if she would know if someone had a disability.

> Depending, depending. I mean if somebody came in with one leg or, you know, something like that ... I would be able to assume possibly that that was considered a disability, but not necessarily.

Interestingly, another nurse manager who worked in a long-term care facility said almost the same thing and laughed as he did so: "I mean if they only had one leg, I'd notice, you know what I mean? I'm not the most observant guy but. ..." This recruiter later amended his original statement regarding not having ever hired anyone with a disability to say: "I can think of several occasions where people had previous back trouble and they did not disclose that and I hired them and it appeared again later.

That has occurred." He went on to explain the ramifications of these types of events.

> I guess I just mean that they didn't volunteer that information. I certainly didn't ask. I would like to think that it doesn't really matter very much to me. You know, if they're doing well enough to try to do this job, then my tendency would be to give them an opportunity to try to do that even if they did disclose it, but they wouldn't tell me because most people would not hire them and they know it. That has worked out well in some occasions and on other occasions it's sorta jumped up and bit me in the butt, worker's comp[ensation] claim and all that stuff.

Nurse managers from long-term care facilities whose patients were predominantly older adults seemed to be the most sympathetic when discussing whether or not a nurse with a disability should be able to work in their facilities. One nurse manager recalled hiring a nurse with a hearing impairment and recalled providing accommodations for that nurse. In cases other than those that involved cognitive disabilities, she felt that nurses with disabilities could be accommodated.

> I think in most settings you can work around a physical disability—perhaps a person would not be able to go and do specific hands-on nursing care but there certainly would be other things within a health care setting that an RN would certainly be able to do that would be helpful to the whole setting. I have never run into a particular case where [for] a person with disabilities we couldn't [find] something for them to do if there was an available position open. You can't create positions for anybody but if there was a position that was open that they had qualifications for, I can't imagine that there wouldn't be some way of coming up with something so that person could do the job.

After having said, this, however, the nurse manager went on to say:

> I've never been in a situation where somebody was physically disabled who has applied and asked for a position who we would have hired. In my millions of years in nursing, I don't ever remember a person with a physical disability, basically hearing impaired yes, physical disability, no, and I'm going back a real long time, being a director of nursing or administrator.

It is likely that in her "millions of years in nursing," a nurse with a physical disability did present her-/himself but hid the disability so well and overcompensated so much that this nurse manager was simply not aware that the nurse had a disability. The amount of energy, both mentally and physically required to hide a disability is significant and wearing over time.

Another nurse manager recalled hiring a nurse with a hearing disability.

> The RN revealed that there were certain bells and all that they could not hear, certain levels or certain tones that they did not hear well. Entering the interview process, we talked about ways that we could accommodate that in this particular unit. And one of the things I did ask this particular RN to do is to disclose always to his coworkers that he does have that disability and that if this person needed to actually work with somebody, they would also be required to help listen for his alarms. That would be something that would be required for him to be able to do to function effectively and safely on the unit.

The manager went on to say that nurses with severely impaired vision or impaired with mobility would not be able to work in her intensive care unit.

Obesity is another issue that can influence whether or not a nurse is hired. Is it a disability? For some institutions and organizations, that seems to be the case. In several of the research studies that were done, nurses self-identified as having a disability rather than having "disability" defined for them. Obesity was considered a disability by a few participants.

One nurse stated that she initially had a phone interview during which everything went well but when she was called in for the in-person interview she was told that she could not have the job. Interestingly, a nurse manager talked about hiring a nurse who was obese and who also had a seizure disorder.

> I hired her knowing these things but talked to her about the necessity of being able to do the job as long as things were under control. Obviously, you know, we could employ her and as long as she could do things that she needed to do with her obesity and all, we could hire her. So we hired her. But over the years—there weren't too many years there—she started having more problems with the seizure, she started having seizures at work. And she reached the point where she couldn't get down on the floor. When a resident falls, you have to get down on the floor to assess them. She couldn't get down on the floor and then get back up [due to her obesity].

It seems clear from the research and anecdotally, that nurses who can hide their disabilities during interviews often do and with good reason.

One manager stated that it was not the policy in any of the places she had worked for many years to provide light duty to nurses who had non work-related physical problems. "If they needed modified duty for walking, that's not work related, they would not provide modified duty for that." She went on to say that depending on the nurse's role, a disability acquired at work would lead to modified duty. She gave examples of jobs a person with a work-related disability could do, such as desk work, "input on the computer, review charts, those kinds of things would help us." However, when asked what would happen if a nurse with a disability was a night supervisor and possibly the only RN in the house, she answered that "perhaps" accommodation might be made. It seems clear that managers may pick and choose for whom they make accommodations.

Another nurse manager echoed this comment but stated that her facility was looking at changing the policy.

> This facility, historically, had not had a light duty, altered job description for a person with a disability or a recent illness or a short-term disability. So, for example, if you came forward and said that "I broke my leg and I can come back to work but I have to be stationary" . . . that has never been permitted. You either come back fully able to do your job description or you did not come back. . . . The current philosophy here is that all nurses manage the essential tasks in their job description and looking at the list of essential tasks, they could not be done if a nurse couldn't speak or hear or be mobile or lift a patient.

One nurse manager summarized the process she and her facility followed when hiring:

> I have hired or interviewed RNs for hire when there was the thought that there might be a disability and what I mean by that is I couldn't tell if it was a temporary disability or a permanent disability. For instance, a nurse walks in that we have made an appointment with by phone and we have already set up an interview and that person might have a limp or be wearing a brace or something else. That's not considered. We don't give any consideration to whether that's a temporary or a permanent disability and obviously we do not ask that and it's not brought up from there. During the interview, we try to find out what the nurse's area of interest is and we attempt to find a unit setting that will be a good fit. It all begins with the job description which identifies the skills necessary to be able to do the job such as being able to lift 50 pounds, turning, squatting, etc. So, if it appears that the person is able to do the job required we send them through the

process and of course they have to pass the physical required by the hospital and after that it is between them and their physician. Now, we have had people call in and inquire and state that they have a specific disability or limitation. At that point, I tell them that we just don't know what might be possible and I encourage them to come in for an interview and see if there is someplace where their skills might be used.

This manager was a rehabilitation nurse and was very committed to "utilizing people with disabilities when we can." This attitude, however was not pervasive among nurse managers or recruiters. More typically, a nurse may have sounded good on the phone or looked good on paper but when they come in for the interview with an obvious disability, attitudes change quickly and usually permanently.

It seems clear from the perceptions of these nurses recruiters and managers that there is some willingness to make accommodations for nurses with disabilities. Yet, most of the recruiters and managers were speaking from a "what if" perspective rather than from experience hiring a nurse they knew had a disability. This presents two interesting points. One is that there do seem to be organizations that are willing to make accommodations and that nurses with disabilities are largely unaware of and unassisted to explore these options. Secondly, the perception by nurse recruiters and nurse managers that they do not recall interviewing anyone with a disability is consistent with the data for nurses with disabilities who say that when they can hide their disabilities, they do so.

THE PERSPECTIVE OF NURSES WITH DISABILITIES

One nurse who had a master's degree, longevity as a nurse, experience as an executive, a manager, and a consultant went to an interview at a teaching hospital. She had hired many nurses herself over the years. Her disability caused her to walk slowly. She told the recruiter that she had been ill and that that explained the gap in her working years but that now she was fine and was returning to work.

> She informed me that it was an extremely stressful job and that she was not quite sure that I could meet the pace that was necessary. [Did] I not get the job because of my disability? I believe so, but I could never prove it.... I exceeded the credentials they were looking for....

This nurse then looked at a case manager position that she could do from home "but they were again concerned about the workload.

You know, there wasn't any incentive on their part to really bring me back." She tried to get other jobs that she could reasonably do. "I tried everything. The thing that got me caught every time was that gap in the work history.... Explaining where it was and why I was not working. By this point, it was 2 years and I eventually stopped because I got sick again...." When this nurse was asked if her experiences had changed the way she felt about nursing, she answered:

> I, unfortunately, have a bad taste in my mouth because we're real caring and accommodating for patients, but we're not for our own peers.... We're supposed to be the ... "helping profession...." Part of the idea is, because you have a disability, you should be willing to take whatever there is, and I don't think that's appropriate.

Another nurse explained

> I just think that people should look at the person for what they can do and not their disability or what they can't do ... to capitalize on their ability and not on their weaknesses. It does not make you feel good to know that you need two good legs or that my vision gets screwed up once in awhile or I forget things. I know these things, no one need tell me these things, but I can sit down and make a phone call and I can assess patients and you know, just look at the person as able, they are able to do this, maybe not THIS, but they can do this.

Another nurse with benign hand tremors admitted to trying to hide her disability during job interviews even though the tremors did not interfere with her work.

> They probably wouldn't have noticed it at the interview.... Unless I have to write something in front of them, they probably wouldn't have noticed it because I keep my hands either together or somehow where they won't notice it.

One nurse educator spoke of her interactions with colleagues regarding her disability and how having a visible disability might have garnered her more help than she actually received.

> I have a fair amount to say about my colleagues. I think this would be true if most people who have what I call an invisible injury so that ... if I came in with an amputation or I came in with something that was visible, I think both the students and ... faculty ...

would [have] a greater awareness of what I'm dealing with. . . . Maybe [every once] in awhile someone will say "How are you doing?" and I'll say "Fine." I could probably say "I'm not doing very well and I wish you'd asked me sooner. . . ." I think much of it has to do with invisibility. The other thing I had noticed . . . is that our university is not handicap friendly. . . . It's very difficult for me to go into the school of nursing building which doesn't have the accessibility. . . . Human Resources actually has been very, very helpful. . . . I tried to find it in the student handbook about disability policy for faculty and they said "We're revising the handbook." . . . so I [went] to the old handbook and as far as I'm concerned it's very inadequate in terms of what it says about illness and disability.

Sometimes, the nursing supervisor or others asked the nurses to hide the disability but most often it was the nurse who chose to hide the disability from others. One nurse with severe allergies said:

The head nurse of the unit . . . said she didn't want me to tell the people that they had perfume on or that I thought they bothered my breathing, because she said I was too blunt and I said OK. So, I said where are you going to be? So, I'd have to go find her, bring her back so she could smell the person . . . and then she'd try to do something about it.

This nurse spoke of the difficulty of having to decide whether to make every nurse in charge aware of the disability so the charge nurse could smell everyone and see if the nurse could take care of that patient or be around that staff person. "We get a super charge nurse practically every shift and so you don't want to disclose your disability, like [you] wear a name badge."

One nurse with a hearing disability verbalized that she wouldn't want to take a job away from another nurse. "If I openly told them, leveled with them, I wouldn't hold it against them because they know what they need." Some nurses with disabilities seem to think they don't deserve to have job choices or to receive accommodations to do a job they can do with their knowledge and skills. They take the approach that they are lucky if they can work as nurses so should be willing to take whatever they are given.

Another nurse with Crohn's disease accepted his limitations and understood that he would need to work part time only and avoid a long commute. He described needing to negotiate and while he had a supportive supervisor, there was "job pressure—the pressure to work more hours, they need you to do more stuff. . . ." He described discussing his disability with his supervisor because they had been peers previously and he knew the supervisor would be understanding. However, this nurse said that he would otherwise hesitate to tell a supervisor about his health issues.

One nurse left traditional nursing for nontraditional nursing work because of the barriers she perceived to nurses with disabilities.

> . . . They would not let you do many things so you hid [the disability] so you tried to do the best you could. In my case, I could hide it. I could literally hide it . . . not to have to let people know it was there. But, there were attitudes regarding people with disabilities. The attitudes that if you had [a] . . . disability you weren't good enough or you couldn't do it or we won't let you do it.

Another nurse spoke of purposely revealing her disability during the interview. "I probably brought it up because usually during an interview they'll say . . . 'Tell me something about yourself that you know might hold you back' . . . That's usually what I tell them."

Another nurse talked about positive responses to her disability. She did not bring it up when she was hired because she didn't think it would affect her work. Most people do not know of her disability unless she tells them "because I try not to make it obvious because I don't like special attention." When asked how others respond when they find out, she said:

> They're fine and most people are helpful, like "Let me carry that for you." The longer I live with it the more accustomed I am to people knowing that I have a disability. So, I am much more open about it these days, but I don't lead with it.

Hiding the disability can be crucial to keeping the job. One nurse worked as a home health nurse in a busy city and in rough neighborhoods. When asked the nature of her disability, she said that it was fatigue that she was able to keep hidden. "[I had to carry] big home health bags and I went in right after the home birth. . . . I would go right in after the baby was delivered and do new baby care and teach. . . ." She also had uneven strength in her arms. When asked if her disability was known when she was first hired she answered:

> . . . At that point, [I] was trying to hide it since this was my dominant arm. I would have carried my bag in my left arm so I just had to [regulate] how I would do things. I can't remember back then if I had let them know or anything that I had a disability because it certainly wasn't something you did back then.

Another nurse who had largely found acceptance in several nursing jobs said this about their current job:

> I don't think people at xxx Mental Health know that I have a disability. I've not had to use a cane. Every once in a while I might be a little stiff when I am standing up and take a couple of wobbly steps and people will look at me funny like what's wrong with you? That would be their first knowledge that I had a disability.

Prior to the latest job, this nurse had worked in orthopedics and attributed the support she had had from colleagues and administrators as being related to their work in orthopedics. This was a similar experience for other orthopedic nurses.

> I think the fact that I was an orthopedic nurse and I was a patient on my working unit, really helped with my coworkers understanding [of] what I was going through and knowing that I was going to have problems with walking and some periods of time when I was going to be uncomfortable. I think if I'd worked in oncology and I'd come back to the oncology unit to work, it might have been a different story. . . . I think if I'd worked on a different unit, the fact that my coworkers had not actually taken care of me post-op in the acute phase of the accident, there would have been disconnect and they might not have been as understanding and accepting. . . . It's like [my colleagues] had been through the accident with me.

One nurse with a latex allergy applied for a job and received a letter of acceptance. During her physical exam, preliminary to beginning the job, she informed the provider that she had the allergy.

> . . . I will never forget, the [health care provider] who was conducting the physical and taking the history, said to me "Well for you to work here, we are going to need a letter from your doctor stating that they can guarantee that you will never have a latex reaction here at the hospital." I just looked at her and you know my heart went down into my toes and stayed there for a very long time. I contacted one of the government agencies that deals with disabilities and they referred me to a local agency in charge of enforcing [ADA rules] and I was told that my case would win in court and that I would be awarded the job. I did not want as a new graduate to begin my career under those circumstances.

This nurse was told about a variety of things she could do to protect herself and still work in patient care, but

> I cannot protect myself from a practitioner who forgets for one moment about the acuity of my allergies and that was my experience in occ[upational] health. I could do everything I might do to protect myself but in one nano second, someone else could place me in jeopardy.

If someone in occupational health could possibly forget that this nurse had latex allergies, then how likely is it that nurses and staff in other settings could remember? Not remembering would place her at great risk. However, there are jobs in nursing that don't involve latex and she was not informed about these jobs.

Another nurse with rheumatoid arthritis who had been at her place of work for more than 20 years said: "I think that my work performance suffered that winter before I was diagnosed. . . . I didn't know what was wrong. . . . I tried to hide a lot of it." When asked how she hid her disability she responded:

> I didn't talk to anybody about anything. I knew that when I came on the unit in the mornings, I'd have to be at work at 5:30, 6 o'clock in the morning. We worked mostly 10 hour shifts And, I would often feel really ill in the morning and I wouldn't complain.

This nurse began to have difficulties she couldn't hide at work.

> In the right hand, [there] was a lot of swelling. I would come in to work and I would literally—sometimes couldn't use one of my hands or I would have difficulty starting an IV and I was treated poorly during that time, knowing that there was something wrong, knowing my coworkers knew that there was a possibility that I had rheumatoid arthritis and in my view I was actually kind of bullied by the manager. . . . Phone calls and the communication that I did have were really directed at: "Well you know, how long are you gonna be out? When are you coming back? Have you been to the doctor? Have you gotten a diagnosis yet?," which in retrospect, I realize that had she known anything about autoimmune diseases, she would know right off the bat that you don't get a diagnosis in 2 days. So, I felt they made me feel as if I was a malingerer and I had a wonderful reputation in this hospital and have always been viewed as someone that had a good work performance, a team player.

It is interesting that there seems to be a phenomenon of labeling nurses who have worked in a setting for a long time, have received good evaluations, and have been highly thought of by their colleagues as malingerers or as not pulling their weight once they become disabled. It is as if none of their previous work mattered anymore. At one point when this nurse was preparing to go back to work after being out due to her illness, her manager called to ask her for

> a list of the things that I could do and couldn't do. When I shared this with the Human Resources Department . . . I remember one of the HR directors rolling her eyes and saying "That's ridiculous, asking you for a list. . . ." Unfortunately, if anybody above [the manager] or around her cared, they didn't come to bat for me.

This nurse later resigned her position.

> I felt as if I couldn't handle the stress of living on the unit any longer and being micro-managed and being watched . . . having no compassion or understanding that I was, indeed sick. . . . I had to make a decision that it was better for me to just get out of this environment.

One nurse with degenerative changes in her spine that caused leg and back pain went back to school to become a nurse practitioner and encountered difficulties in her clinical practica. The nurse had problems caring for totally dependent patients in a skilled nursing facility and in bending down to inspect the feet of diabetic patients. Her preceptors asked: "Well, how are you going to be a nurse practitioner if you can't do this?" The nurse responded

> I'm not going to be working at a nursing facility, I'm going to work in a doctor's office. And if I can't find a place, I'm going to wait until I find a place. So, that is my choice. . . . [The preceptor] kind of had a strange attitude about it and . . . I kind of had to disclose [the disability] because it is clearly visible. . . .

This nurse became a nurse practitioner and had been applying for jobs at the time of the research interview.

> So, I do not plan on telling my employer that I suffer from depression. I may or may not tell them that I have fibromyalgia and I probably will tell them that I have a herniated disc. . . . It shouldn't be an issue because the pain doesn't really have [anything] to do [with] an office environment.

One nurse who has partial paralysis of one leg and uses a crutch to assist her to walk described good experiences going through nursing school despite her disability. Initially, she was also pleased with the responses of others when she went to work.

> Up until a few weeks ago, it was like a fairy tale. I just felt like I was everyone's best friend and everyone was mine and it went fantastic and everyone was supportive and as much as they would give to me, I would give back and I did precepting for students a lot and I never knew that what I thought I was giving to the unit by precepting a few people [was viewed as she] always has help. Thinking that I had help versus thinking that I was trying to teach which is ultimately what I want to do. . . .

This nurse's impulse to teach other nurses was met with suspicion because she had a disability. It doesn't seem likely that if she didn't have a disability others would be so quick to interpret her motives as self-serving rather than as selfless.

Another nurse who needs to use a cane discussed her experiences trying to get hired:

> I was very explicit in the fact that I had knee problems and why I limped and why I use a cane and why I used a walker, figuring it's better to be honest right up front so that they knew what they were getting into if they hired me. And they would say "Oh, that's no problem" and then I would never hear from them again . . . (Neal-Boylan, 2012). They send me a proverbial letter stating "We have no positions at this time" or they don't respond at all, and that's what happens most of the time. I explicitly tell the person [with whom] I am interviewing "I can do my job. It may take me a couple minutes longer, but I can do my job." [They] don't care.

This nurse continued by describing what then happened four months after being hired in an inpatient job:

> They started giving me grief because I was too slow in getting to emergencies from one side of the building to the other. . . . It took me maybe three to four minutes to get from one side of the building to another and I was able to deal with the emergencies, no sweat, but they were giving me more grief. They were gonna fire me because I didn't tell them, supposedly, that I had a disability.

Another nurse with arthritis in multiple joints talked about applying for a job with hospice.

> Hospice needed nurses desperately, and I gave [them] my résumé and they loved it. They thought it was wonderful. They called me right up. [They asked me to] "Please come right over. . . ." [In the interview], I am sitting down [and] I look like I'm perfectly normal. You'd never know. And then, as I stood up, well they shake hands with you [so you] need to stand up, so I could see the face just go ugh! They see my posture . . . they just see a worker's compensation case. I can see it in their face right now. I should just turned around and left then. They are obligated though, they've known, 'cause of discrimination law suits, they have to interview me . . . and almost every single [job] has given me a second interview, just to make sure I don't file anything.

This nurse offered to be precepted and offered to work for very little money to start with. She suggested that someone go out on a home hospice visit with her,

> and at the end of that time, I said, you can check me over, see if I'm able to go out and do home cases myself or not. . . . I said there's no obligation on either [side]; you don't have to [give me] benefits, you don't have to do anything but it's helping me and at the same time, you're getting an RN. . . . They didn't even call me back. I wrote them a repeat letter back, saying I didn't know if [they received] my first letter, I just wanted to do a follow up and nothing . . . nothing.

The nurse continued to apply for jobs in home care because the home health agencies were desperate for nurses. Then, because of her experience in psychiatric mental health nursing a manager of psychiatric nursing in a home care agency called her saying "Would you mind, we really need nurses in . . . psych home care right now."

> I go over there, and again, sitting down, I'm fine. The minute I stand up, the lady's face, I can see it. . . . I could tell the receptionist, as soon as I came and told her who I was and what I was interviewing for . . . she got on the phone. I could hear whispering behind me. I think she was calling this lady to tell her . . . that hey, you don't want this one. . . .

When the receptionist prepared to take the nurse upstairs for the interview, the receptionist suggested that they take the elevator, saying "I don't know if you can do the stairs." The nurse answered: "I have no problem doing stairs. . . . If you like, I'll be happy to do them with you."

She made me do the elevator. We did that. I think I had the world's quickest interview—2 minutes flat. Then she actually had the audacity to take my elbow and hold my arm as I walked out of there, to meet me downstairs to get me out of the building. . . . I left there in tears.

Another nurse said:

I would look good on paper and during the phone interview and I would get there and they would come around the corner, they would see the crutch and you could just kind of see that glaze over in their eyes like, uh oh, what do I do now?

When asked if any of the jobs for which she had applied stopped the interview process as soon as they saw that she had a disability, she answered:

No, they all went through with the interview but one job in particular, I knew how many candidates they had and how many job openings there were and we had talked very freely about it and I thought it was a slam dunk in the bag and the next thing I know they have an extended interview process and I just sat there feeling very sad because disabilities can make you question yourself, your worthiness, am I being a burden on other people, and a lot of times, you feel that way more with your family so when you are in the work place and you are feeling that pride and you're feeling that I am a nurse and I am making a difference, you don't want someone to look at you like you are not worthy of a job, especially during a nursing shortage.

One nurse with a disability began to work in private duty home care because she thought she could manage the work load and the hours and was asked to take on a patient who was in a coma and was tube fed and also had a urinary catheter. Her supervisor was trying hard to give her clinical work.

. . . But this is part of the problem. The most difficult thing about trying to work with a disability. . . . She said to me while we were [in the patient's home], she said "Well, gee, maybe this might be a good place . . . for you to do some hours." First of all, I was thinking right off the bat, I was surprised that she would pick someone like that and thinking that that would be a good fit for me. . . . She didn't see that I was limping. She didn't know. . . . I'm damned if

I do, and damned if I don't. If I complain, what do I look like? ... How do you come across when you complain? And on the other hand, if I don't complain, people look at me and think I'm fine. ... In my mind, I'm thinking "Oh God, it's like I have to fight so many battles on so many levels with this thing. What is she thinking?"

One nurse with a chronic debilitating disease expressed his feelings this way:

I like people to have some other view of me before that's the first thing they see. Which I think is a fairly universal thought about disabilities. . . . You don't want to be the disability. You don't want to be . . . YOU, the person in the wheelchair, you're the person with diabetes . . . you are the disability. But that's not your whole identity.

Yet, some nurses think that having a visible or obvious disability can make it easier to get the help the nurse needs to do his or her job. One nurse said:

. . . I think people are more sympathetic towards a disability when they can actually see somebody limping or they see a limb that's missing. I think people that have disabilities for nonvisible reasons have a much harder time with understanding from their peers than we have [with] a visible disability.

Most nurses with disabilities do try to hide them if possible for fear of repercussions. As one nurse explained: "I was afraid that they would decide that I was not a useful member of the team if I admitted to having any frailty and so it was really something I didn't talk about because I didn't want it to be a whole mess" (Neal-Boylan & Guillett, 2088a, 2008b, 2008c).

Other nurses say that having a nurse in some jobs is sufficient and that there is little concern over what the nurse can or cannot do until she or he begins the job. A school nurse said:

I think that when you interview for a job, when you're disabled, you don't realize until it really happens to you. You really don't want to go over and over about this disability. You try to compensate for what you can't do but I think they should have a job description. It's almost like, well, we need a nurse in school otherwise we're not gonna get state funding so we're gonna use you and that's the attitude I get. They don't even think to ask are you physically able to do this. They just assume that if you're coming for this job, you can physically do it but there is no real job description.

A nurse with rheumatoid arthritis felt that she had been pushed out of her previous job so did not discuss her diagnosis in a subsequent job interview. ".... When I went for the interview [of] course I never talk about my diagnosis, so I got the job there." The nurse had trouble handling the few steps that she needed to navigate during her work day. "... I can handle the step but I don't do it like normal. I don't know if they picked up on that or what." "They" probably meaning the nurse manager. She began learning the job, was able to do it and came to enjoy it.

So I was doing okay and then after a few weeks, [the manager] started giving me a hard time about things. I was just so new, it was less than a month and she started sorta picking on me in a way that I couldn't figure out. I never experienced anything like that before.

SOLUTIONS

It is clear that nurses with disabilities often hide their disabilities, when possible. It is not hard to understand why, given some of the experiences of nurses who have revealed their disabilities. Interestingly, nurse recruiters and managers often could not recall interviewing a nurse with a disability although some acknowledged working with nurses who acquired disabilities on the job. Why should there be such a disconnect? The nursing profession is filled with a variety of jobs and positions that don't require physical strength or endurance. Some can be done even if the nurse has difficulty verbally communicating. Others can be performed with a hearing disability. There may be others that could be done using Braille for a nurse who cannot see.

There is a major contraindication between what we say as a profession—that we want to be valued for our intellect, critical thinking skills, expertise, and ability to make quick but sound judgments—and how we view ourselves in reality. Nurses appear to look down on each other and if one nurse is not able to function perfectly, there appears to be little in the way of empathy or support. Nurses on orthopedic floors tend to be the exception when it comes to musculoskeletal disabilities. There are also isolated instances of compassion and tolerance and sincere attempts to help a nurse with a disability do his or her work. On the whole, though, both the research data and anecdotal comments from nurses with disabilities indicate that both subtle and obvious displays of discrimination occur.

Nurses with disabilities, for the most part, seem to know that they are not suited to all types of nursing and appear understanding regarding the need, on occasion, to move them to other areas of nursing better suited to their ability to function effectively despite the disability. Nurses don't want to jeopardize patient safety. They don't like not being able to pull their weight or letting down their colleagues. The problem is that an inability to function the way everyone else might be able to function is viewed as letting others down, such as in the cases of nurses whose fatigue prevents them from working nights or full time. Perhaps if nurses viewed their colleagues with disabilities as they might view patients they would have more compassion for them. This is not to suggest that nurses with disabilities should be treated differently, only that they should receive the same consideration and compassion that a nurse would give someone who was a patient instead of a colleague and had a disability. It has often been said that nurses eat their young. It appears that they also eat each other. As the nursing workforce continues to age, the likelihood of disability grows. We cannot discard or afford to lose nurses with disabilities.

If nurses with disabilities were made to feel that they were not automatically discounted as potential employees or that there was some consideration given to jobs that they could do within the health care organization, they might be less inclined to hide their disabilities from nurse recruiters and nurse managers. As a nurse with disabilities said:

> ... Maybe when they are going over the laws regarding not discriminating [recruiters could] talk about the fact that when you are busy not discriminating, don't forget to look at the person and to talk to the person and be open and to hear what they have to say because I remember this one person I interviewed for. I said, I understand that you could look at me and think that I might not be able to do the physical rigors of this job, but why don't we go over there and I'll show you what I can do and she said, "Oh no, no, no, you don't have to worry about that." I never got the opportunity and it was really sad.

Conversely, nurse managers and recruiters should adopt a demeanor that signifies openness to the possibilities of having a nurse with a disability work in their organizations. Efforts should be made to discuss the actual work of the job rather than to continue to depend on the traditional nurse job descriptions that so often mandate certain lifting requirements and other physical abilities even when the job may not actually require them. Could a nurse's aide realistically assist the nurse or perform the physical care required? How often, in actuality, does the nurse really need to lift the patient or otherwise perform physical tasks? Can accommodations be made without exorbitant expense? Is the cost worth it if the organization can hire qualified nurses and retain them? How much does the organization and nursing risk losing when we do not hire or make the effort to retain a nurse with a disability?

These are questions that demand answers if we are to retain nurses with disabilities. Nursing is a tradition-based profession while also being scientifically based and proud of it. Consequently, we should be able to pride ourselves in being able to change the way we have always done things by looking at each job individually and carefully to determine what actually is required to perform it effectively and if there are ways a nurse with a disability could be accommodated so he or she could do the job.

REFERENCES

Neal-Boylan, L. J. (2012). An exploration and comparison of the worklife experiences of registered nurses and physicians with permanent physical and/or sensory disabilities. *Rehabilitation Nursing, 37*(1), 3–10.

Neal-Boylan, L. J., & Guillett, S. E. (2008a). Nurses with disabilities: Can changing our educational system keep them in nursing? *Nurse Educator, 33*(4), 1–4.

Neal-Boylan, L. J., & Guillett, S. E. (2008b). Registered nurses with physical disabilities. *Journal of Nursing Administration, 38*(1), 1–3.

Neal-Boylan, L. J., & Guillett, S. E. (2008c). Work experiences of RNs with physical disabilities. *Rehabilitation Nursing, 33*(2), 67–72.

Neal-Boylan, L. J., Hopkins, A., Skeete, R., Hartmann, S. B., Iezzoni, L. I., & Nunez-Smith, M. (2012). The career trajectories of health care professionals practicing with permanent disabilities. *Academic Medicine, 87*(2), 172–178.

BIBLIOGRAPHY

Guillett, S. E., Neal-Boylan, L. J., & Lathrop, R. (2007). Ready, willing, and disabled. *American Nurse Today, 2*(8), 30–32.

Neal-Boylan, L. J., Fennie, K., & Baldauf-Wagner, S. (2011). Nurses with sensory disabilities: Their perceptions and characteristics. *Rehabilitation Nursing, 36*(1), 25–31.

4
Disability, Job Longevity, and Career Choice

Natalie, a 35-year-old registered nurse with multiple sclerosis, worked on an orthopedic floor for several years. Her condition was gradually progressive so she was able to manage quite well for a long time and the orthopedic nurses were particularly understanding regarding her symptoms as they were used to working with patients with chronic disease. Eventually, however, it became more difficult for Natalie to walk up and down the long hallways, to move and lift patients, and to work long shifts. She was also getting sick more frequently than previously. Despite having worked at the facility for several years, she still had to take evening and night shifts on occasion and float to other units. Natalie felt that the time had come for her to find a less physically demanding job. She decided to interview for a home care position. She got the job and was expected to see an average of eight patients each day. She did not mind the driving as she found that she could usually travel at her own pace and take breaks when she needed them. She liked the idea of being able to see her patients in their own environments and to be able to view their care holistically. Over time, she got to know many of her patients well and enjoyed interacting with them. Seeing eight patients a day, however, was difficult. By this time, Natalie needed to use a cane and climbing stairs into apartments required extra time. At one point, her manager called her into the field office and told her that her productivity was not sufficient and that she needed to increase the number of patients she was seeing. Natalie explained that she was trying very hard but could not manage that. She asked to be able to cut down to 4 days a week and have a fifth day off in the middle of the week so she could have a rest day. Natalie felt that she would then have a better chance of increasing her productivity during the days she was at work but didn't feel she could promise to see eight patients a day. The manager said that she could not provide this position. Natalie was very disappointed but realized that if she became too fatigued she was likely to cause a relapse in her condition. She switched to another home care agency that included private duty home care as well as intermittent skilled

> nursing visits. Natalie was able to do 8-hour day-shifts caring for one patient in the patient's home. This worked well, because the patient's wife was able to help lift and move the patient and Natalie was able to sit for a good deal of her shift. However, because of being immunosuppressed from multiple sclerosis, Natalie found that she was increasingly vulnerable to illness. She had to leave this job but eventually found work as an advice nurse and case manager for a large health insurance company. She grieved over having to leave direct patient care and felt that accommodations could have been made that would have enabled her to continue to work with patients but she was unable to get any guidance or any support to do this.

Some nurses with disabilities are disabled before they begin working in nursing, others become disabled once they are nurses. In either case, however, the nurse is often confronted with the need to make career and job choices because he or she has a disability. Sometimes, the nurse cannot find a job at all, despite acknowledged nursing experience and expertise. This chapter will discuss the job and career choices nurses with disabilities make when they recognize that they can't work in the job in which they have been working or in their ideal job. As this book has so far discussed, sometimes the nurse chooses to leave the job but more often, the nurse feels pushed out of the job for reasons related to having a disability. Often, the choice to leave the job or nursing altogether leads to serious financial problems and difficulties at home. As one nurse said:

> [I've] not been able to work. I've run into financial difficulties and right now I'm filing bankruptcy because I should not work. My husband's unemployed, he gets a pension, and what are we gonna do? How are we going to pay for my house and stay here? I am at risk of foreclosure at this moment. . . . I wanna stay here but how can I if and when I can't work? My salary every week was enough to get us by with my husband's social security and pension plan to pay all of our bills and my mortgage. I can't do that anymore, seeing that nobody will hire me when I walk in for an interview.

This nurse sought legal counsel to get help. She was turned down for various reasons.

> Then I went to a second attorney for an appeal . . . the attorney said I would win my case and then it was a matter of coming up with a retainer for his fees. Then he said, once he learned we were

filing bankruptcy, "forget it." He wasn't going to take it. . . . So I'm left out in the cold.

This nurse had 40 years of nursing experience at the time of the research interview. "I feel confident enough. I can do anything, practically." She needed to use a cane or a walker to get from place to place. Despite her disability, she had at one time been a night supervisor in long-term care for the whole building. She felt that she was seen as a liability by management and that that was why she couldn't get a nursing position. "They see it as a liability, more than a minor interference in me getting around and being able to do my job, where I could do it very well. They didn't see it that way." This nurse had multiple jobs and perceived that she was let go because of her disability and not from an inability to do her job well. Most frequently, administrators do not appear to make any effort to help the nurse or to find ways to retain the nurse within the organization by offering another position.

> Nobody has ever asked me "What can we do as management to make your performance easier or make it better so that we can help you to make our facility and/or plan of action for patient care better." Nobody.

At one point, this nurse made a change to private duty home care caring for a very ill child. This worked very well for her.

> [The mother] needed to sleep and she was happier than Hades that I was there and she could sleep at night and she felt very capable that I was there and I was able to take care of her daughter and if and when there were any questions, I would wake her up and ask specific questions and her input into the care of her daughter.

The change to home care seemed reasonable because the nurse could work nights. She also enjoyed the private duty work.

> It gave me greater satisfaction to see immediate results and what I did for the patient. A better rapport with the family and immediate interaction with the family if any problems came up and we could co-solve the problem together and come up with a solution for the betterment of the welfare of the child. Because [of] the interaction I had with the daughter and with the mother, we had bonded. We would talk about how the child had changed and what transpired during the night and what I did to relieve any

problems if there were any, and I would consult her immediately if there were problems and she was perfectly satisfied with my services.

When the nurse could no longer see this patient because having a disability affected her ability to pass her cardiopulmonary resuscitation (CPR) test, the mother of the baby became very upset when she heard the news. As for the nurse, she had had enough.

I just want out of nursing.... [I have] disillusionment with the profession itself. There's a saying out there that they-we eat our own and they do. Because my friends and I discuss this frequently when we get together, of attitudes, management, decisions, experiences we all go through. Inevitably, we all come to [the] conclusion: All of our experiences are similar in nature and the results are very similar in nature.... I'm scared because I don't have a paycheck coming in. I'm scared because I may lose my house and where the hell am I gonna go? What am I gonna do?

Difficulty with CPR and passing the test was a fairly common theme for nurses with musculoskeletal disabilities and reduced strength. Is it necessary, in the age of portable defibrillators, for all nurses to be able to do CPR, regardless of their place of work? Isn't the use of the defibrillator more significant in saving lives from cardiac arrest than is the ability to perform CPR? The nurse is still capable of assessing the situation, pinpointing what is needed, initiating defibrillator use, calling 911, and mobilizing emergency resources. Should the inability to perform CPR, by itself, prevent a nurse from working as a nurse? The correct answer is that it depends on the setting and the acuity of the patients. Naturally, if a nurse could not perform CPR, there are settings in which she or he should not work. However, there may be instances in which other strategies might work just as well or even better than having a nurse perform CPR.

TRYING TO FIT IN SOMEWHERE

Nurses with disabilities often have difficulty finding a job that they have the expertise and skills to do and can also physically accomplish. Sometimes, employers have good intentions and try to find a job the nurse can do but they are not always completely aware of all of the aspects of the situation. One nurse with an autoimmune disease that affected her ability to function physically made the move to private duty home care. After revealing her disability, she was told "We can work this out. We can find a case that's a light case and you could do 4 hour blocks instead of an 8 hour day." However, she was assigned cases that because of their high acuity and risk of infection, put her at high risk and were difficult for her to manage.

> I'm not sure we have long enough for me to convey what I went through over the last 2 years, trying to get back to work, trying to find a place in society where I can function well and have all these talents, and I can't fit in anywhere.

This nurse spoke of her thought processes and considerations when she was looking for a job that she could do.

> How do I have to use my body for this job? I considered working in book stores. I considered working in food service, but I would have to, every time I thought about a job, I would have to think about my body and I would have to imagine a shift or a day and what I would be doing. Would I be standing all day in the same place? . . . [I] can't sit all day. [I] can't do repetitive motions all day. . . . And then, of course, the other issues. I mean . . . is it worth it to go work for $8 an hour and ultimately down the road, after nine months, lose my disability? Is it worth it? But I was looking at $8 an hour jobs 'cause I wanted to work somewhere so much that at one point, I would have done that. Those were the main stumbling blocks for me: physical limitations and the environment that I would be exposed to, in terms of being immunosuppressed.

So many nurses with disabilities simply love nursing and want to stay in the profession, even if it means that they are not able to pursue their specific passion. They are often willing to do anything that involves nursing. It does not seem unreasonable, given the frequent nursing shortages and the various types of nursing, for a nurse with disabilities to be able to continue to work as a nurse.

Another nurse also tried to work in home care but had trouble getting past the interview once people saw that she was disabled. So, she applied for a position at Planned Parenthood. She met with people there several times but they did not, at first, give her a job. But the nurse recruiter told her that they really liked her and asked if she would consider working there per diem. She agreed, went through orientation and was working on and off for them at the time of the research interview. She was grateful for the work, but working per diem made her work schedule irregular and unpredictable. Another nurse discussed the lack of support from administrators regarding trying to find an alternative to the current job.

I was very well known. I'd been there for a long time and [was] very well respected and there was a fair level of awareness that I was going through this at the time but there wasn't any attempt from any level to help me out. I tend not to be a fighter and so maybe I should have made more of an issue. Maybe I should have become more assertive and more proactive. The mistake that I made, and even to this day, I kind of regret it, is making that decision to leave. I left there and went to another job. I didn't want to stop working at that point. . . . I was already spending a lot of time reevaluating where I was going to work and I had been feeling very frustrated with mainstream health care and I was getting very frustrated with the hospital environment even though this was a hospital I knew well and felt that it was home in a lot of ways. So, I was feeling a lot of that but after I got sick, literally I was concerned about if I continue on with these symptoms, will I be able to do what's required of me? And, secondly, I really felt so threatened and really wounded by the way I was treated after being such a valuable employee that . . . there was no one supporting me.

This nurse went from the hospital to a private practice. "They were thrilled to have me." The nurse revealed her disability and the work went well until the practice later lost its physician.

Another nurse with musculoskeletal difficulties from an autoimmune disease worked quite happily as a school nurse until she was hit with her diagnosis. She had been working at a handicapped accessible school because a lot of the children at the school were in wheelchairs. After her diagnosis and having been at that school for more than 10 years, she was reassigned to another school.

They were two smaller schools, very old buildings, not handicap accessible, both health rooms were on the second floor so I had to climb flights of stairs to get to the health room. I never told them my diagnosis but they knew I had a physical problem in that way even though, at that point, I didn't think it was compromising my ability to do the job. Many days, I went to work in pain and just sort of pushed through. . . . Because of my disability, they got rid of me. At that time, I felt like I could still do the job or was going to try to do the job. If I had decided I wasn't capable of it, I would have left, you know? It wasn't discussed with me. [No one said] "Well, what if we do this for you . . ." but they purposely put me in a school where it was very difficult physically. . . . So after that, well, that was devastating, absolutely devastating for me.

This nurse decided to go to the labor board and complain and although her union representative was not available to her, she knew someone who worked for the state and was able to get a retired union representative to go with her to the hearing.

> She didn't have to work very hard 'cause it was just so blatant what they had done.... I'd never experienced anything like that, I didn't know what to expect, it was terrible. It was humiliating. But that's one thing about this disability and employment, it becomes a very humiliating experience.

The nurse won the case and was able to collect unemployment benefits. She was told by her attorney that she could fight for her job and get it back but by that time "I felt like I didn't want to work for those people anymore."

> Now, after that, I had to deal with trying to get another job. And the uncomfortable feeling when you apply ... and you have to put down that you were terminated. Well, right there is a red flag for an employer, let's face it. So, I felt like that really did a lot of damage to my reputation and my work record, my employment history. Prior to that, I never ever had a problem whenever I applied for a job, I always got the job and now this became much more challenging as a result of this.

Ultimately, the nurse got a job working at another school.

> That's when I came to the realization [that] I had to go out to the [playing] field for emergencies and it was very difficult.... [After a few months] I had decided that I could no longer do this job. I made a decision that the liability was too great. So I resigned from there.

She went on to get a job in an outpatient clinic. She relearned skills that she hadn't used in the many years of school nursing. She enjoyed it and all appeared to be going well. After less than a month on the job, she was reprimanded because of the way she opened a box.

> ... a little teeny box. Well, I got a lecture about how I opened the box. I didn't open it correctly.... I never really gave it much thought before. I never ever had a discussion about opening the box with any peer.... So, that's when [the supervisor] started giving me a hard time for different things.... It wasn't really my

nursing. She really couldn't go after that, because I was doing well. It was all this picky stuff. I thought perhaps she could see that I had some difficulty walking.

Another school nurse described school nursing as being a place for a nurse with a disability to work, depending on the disability.

Yes, it depends on the disability. . . . Because it forces you to see if you can really do things. . . . If there's a trauma, you're calling 911, you may have to start CPR. . . . If I had to get down and do CPR, I would be able to get down on the floor but to be able to jump back up right away, that's where my disability would come in. I wouldn't be able to get up quickly.

This school nurse did not feel that her disability precluded her from working in a hospital setting but did have concerns about how she might handle a patient who had fallen if she was working in a hospital and was alone.

I always have my cell phone on me, where I could call 911 and I would yell for help, but I think if people are gonna go into a nursing situation, you think about what you do as a nurse because I could go back into a hospital. It's not that they won't hire me, but I'm thinking well, if I'm in a situation how do I handle this and there's nobody around. . . . But . . . there's less of a chance of something like that happening as a school nurse than there is as a hospital nurse.

One nurse who had difficulties with her hands admitted:

I love surgery but I don't think I would ever work in the OR [operating room] because of [my hands]. Unless it's just circulating, I would circulate without a problem. I don't like to scrub just for the reason I don't wanna knock anything off. . . . I have no fine motor skills whatsoever. (Neal-Boylan, 2012)

She made a conscious decision regarding what kind of nursing she would do because of her hands.

But I didn't know it was gonna get this bad either. If I had known they were gonna be this bad, I might not have even gone into nursing at all. I don't know . . . and it actually makes me want to get out of the patient care aspect of nursing more and get into maybe the paperwork aspect more, somewhere. I've thought about being a nurse consultant . . . or even working for an insurance company. . . . I mean that's not where I wanna be, that's not where I wanna put my nursing skills but at some point that may be where I have to be. . . . Oh, I love this job. I'd stay here as long as I could. Definitely. . . . I like the happy times. . . .

Contract work seems like a common alternative for some nurses with disabilities. Fatigue guides many of the job choices nurses make. Careful consideration must occur for those nurses who are on long-term disability as they might lose the benefits depending on the number of hours they work or the money they make.

Volunteer work is an alternative that uses the nurse's skills but allows them flexibility and the option to not work if they don't feel physically able. One nurse talked about volunteering for the American Red Cross "and they are extremely accommodating." She told the people who offered her a volunteer position about her disability and they told her that that was not a problem. "So they want me on their disaster team. . . . I'm gonna be teaching for them and I can't teach all day so a class that's 8 hours, I can split up any way I want."

If the American Red Cross recognizes that having a trained nurse with solid nursing experience is worth accommodating work hours for, then why is this not possible for organizations that provide paying jobs? Couldn't a nurse with a disability be hired to teach health education classes or perform work that can be scheduled for a few hours at a time and not require prolonged standing or activity? Certainly, this would not apply to all or even most nursing jobs, but surely there are jobs that can be tailored to suit nurses with disabilities and for which they can be paid.

A nurse who had been an administrator for many years was no longer being utilized in that position because of her disability. She left the job voluntarily but had hoped that she would be brought back in some capacity. "I have had experience and a lot of it, my knowledge should be utilized more so patients and people can benefit from my good nursing practice." She also felt that she could be used as a consultant ". . . telephonically, I could give them instructions and help them know how to do things. . . . They need knowledge. . . . I can help others because my knowledge is great and it needs to be shared."

ABILITY TO DO THE WORK

Many nurses are able to cut their shifts to allow them to continue to work. One nurse originally worked 12-hour shifts and was able to cut them to 4-hour shifts. This nurse had worked at the same institution for almost

20 years and felt that that had a lot to do with the facility's willingness to accommodate him. He had arthritis and hearing loss and commented that he didn't think he could work on the floor in the hospital because of the large number of patients for which each nurse was responsible. This nurse worked in critical care and liked the fact that he worked in a small space with fewer patients but he recognized that not all nurses with disabilities could or would necessarily want to stay at the bedside. "There's many things you can do besides bedside [care]. In fact, nowadays, most nurses don't want to stay at the bedside that long. They want to get an advanced degree or do something else."

This nurse had had to make some of his own accommodations to be able to stay in critical care

> . . . because it's hard to drown out the noise from the other communication whereas supposedly they're making hearing aids now that [do] that. . . . You really have [to] sometimes . . . ask them to speak louder, say to doctors. You really have to pay attention or you ask them . . . write it down, don't just tell [me] 'cause that way there's no mix up.

Another nurse with mobility issues started looking at her options when she realized that she could no longer run down hospital hallways. She examined which skills she had that were transferable to other settings. She was a master's prepared nurse with more than 20 years in nursing with experience as an executive, administrator, and consultant. She applied for over a hundred jobs. Not one of the employers from whom she had applied for a job in nursing offered her any explanation regarding why they would not offer her a job. She tried to go into teaching but did not have recent clinical experience, only managerial and consultant experience, so was not hired. She started lobbying for the rights of people with disabilities in her state. She also decided to get a second graduate degree.

> There doesn't seem to be a niche for nurses that are disabled. You know if we go back, it's usually to a much lower paying position that we may not want to be in but it's the only way that they can accommodate us. . . . As nursing expands as a profession, I can think of a lot of arenas where whatever disability you have could be accommodated.

However, this nurse also commented that a nurse with a disability should not have to resign him-/herself to accept a job that they don't want or to have to start at the beginning again when they have been in nursing for a long time.

> The job opportunities are prohibitive. I could probably go back on a part-time basis at a staff level. I haven't been staff level in 20 years. . . . It's self-actualization, it's self-assurance, it's confidence. And you know, if you're in something that is not building that, you don't want to get up every morning and go. . . . Nobody would want to do that, disabled or able. Let's be real.

Her work lobbying for the rights of people with disabilities and experience working in health insurance led her to mount a letter-writing campaign to her legislators. She felt that what she had experienced and what others with disabilities had experienced was the result of discrimination. As a result of her efforts, she was able to change the law in her state regarding disabled individuals. She did not feel that the Americans with Disabilities Act (ADA) had significantly helped people with disabilities because so many disabilities are not visible.

> Disabilities come in many shapes, sizes, and forms. Not being in a wheelchair doesn't mean that you're not disabled . . . because people will look at you when you get out of your car with disabled tags on and say "You look okay to me." It's not always what you can see. . . . So the ADA has not helped us.

Her solution to her own difficulties with getting a job in nursing was to get a second graduate degree and start her own practice. She was able to take most of her courses online from home.

GOING BACK TO SCHOOL: TO WORK OR LEARN

It is not uncommon for nurses with disabilities to become creative about carving a niche for themselves in nursing and many go back to school for more education. This often takes them further from the bedside but those who become advanced practice nurses (APN) still care for patients but on their own terms and with less physical labor than they might have had in other settings. In many private practices and in community clinics, an APN often has a medical or nursing assistant who takes the vital signs, weighs the patient, and puts the patient in a room. The APN in primary care does not typically perform any physical activity that would require strength or endurance. The APN is acknowledged to be employed because of his or her advanced level of expertise and critical thinking.

The APN assesses the patient and makes diagnoses and prescribes treatment. This kind of role has been very well suited to nurses with disabilities. Why is it hard to understand then how a registered nurse in an inpatient setting, for example, could rely on others for the physical care and movement of the patient? The registered nurse is still expected to assess the patient and carry out the orders of the APN, physician, or physician's assistant. The nurse with a disability is likely to be no less capable of doing so and implementing care because of the disability as long as she or he is still able to think critically and use his or her expertise to manage and alter the plan of care.

So much may depend on the setting in which the registered nurse or APN works. One nurse practitioner, with pain and reduced function in multiple joints, had previously done consultation work in an assisted living facility. She previously had seen almost 20 patients each day but could no longer manage that volume. This nurse had started out in staff nursing and after hurting her back lifting a patient, a fall, and a car accident, she realized that her best option was to return to school. When she could no longer walk the floors at the assisted living facility or manage the high volume of patients, she went into private practice where she could manage her own hours and work load. She also taught clinicals for nursing students and was in a setting that allowed her to sit often.

> I have always had an optimistic attitude. I've been flexible and resilient. So if something happens to me, it's not the end of the world. I'm going to find something else. It's just my personality. Other people I know say, "Well, this is it, I'm gonna go on disability," but I wore a cast on my hand for 2 years and had pins and screws and I walked around the floors with students like the Statue of Liberty. I did that for 2 years when I said I could stay home, but I want to be with students so here I was.

Should only nurses with optimistic attitudes, flexibility, and resilience be able to find jobs in nursing? Is it fair for the nurse with a disability to have to work so hard to even find a job when the nurse is potentially already coping with pain and fatigue? It seems possible that nursing, as a profession could make it easier for nurses with disabilities to find jobs within their organizations or to move to other jobs in which they could use their abilities rather than having to give up on nursing. Perhaps a nationwide database could be developed that would highlight jobs that are available for nurses with disabilities.

A nurse with hand tremors consciously made the decision not to go back to school to become a nurse educator.

> I would never want to be an instructor 'cause I couldn't show them how to do it correctly. I [could] not be sure I wasn't contaminating something.... You have to be very precise and show them the

exact way. Whether it's done like that in the real world or not, that's the way it's supposed to be done.

Some nurses with disabilities go into school nursing if there are no difficulties getting into or around in the school.

> It took me a year of looking around before I found something that was going to work, both that I wanted to do and that the hours and the timing and location that would all work out so that's how I ended up working in the schools.... It's pretty much 30 hours a week and they're not always saying, "Well, we have this other site you need to cover and can you just work another shift." It's close to home so there isn't, on top of however many hours of working days, a couple of hours of driving time. So, it really is 30 hours, which the difference in how much energy I have at that point is very big. So far, so good.... I essentially have the summer off because it's a school, it's on a school calendar and so I did per diem work over the summer.... I'd work for years per diem, not per diem, but what's called a flat position which means that it could be any days, any hours. It added up to the same number of hours, more or less, in a 2-week period.... One time I could be working at 8 in the morning, another time I could be working till 8 or 9 at night. So, it's like shifts in the hospital where you work one shift and then you work another shift, and that's also very hard to adapt to, for anybody.... It only took me 6 years to get to the point of figuring out that I couldn't be doing that anymore.

CHANGING CAREER GOALS

Nurses with disabilities frequently have to reassess what they see as their professional future, given their disabilities. Can they stay in nursing and find something that will excite them? Should they leave nursing and explore other fields that might be more empathetic to someone with a disability? It is a very tough choice, especially considering that nurses are given very little formalized assistance regarding their options for staying in nursing.

A nurse with a latex allergy was forced to change her career goals once she was aware that she had the allergy.

> I wanted to immediately enroll in a program to become a CRNA (certified registered nurse anesthetist) and I was unable to do so.... I did try briefly, probably against advice, to practice in an

occupational health setting and my allergist ... basically said "Well, obviously you have made peace with the idea of dying from your latex allergy. . . ." And that really gave me pause and I left that position after a very brief period of time.

This nurse moved into health policy and "was very successful . . . but I could tell you my first love and true passion depends on patient care." She expressed concern that nurses with disabilities have such a hard time being valued for their abilities.

I think that many organizations are unable to look beyond the skill set that an individual brings. They are truly viewed totally and solely in terms of their disability and the potential liability that it might bring and that is such a tragedy.

Often nurses leave a bedside nursing position and intentionally seek and find a position that allows them to remain in nursing and does not require them to exert themselves physically. These nurses take desk jobs, positions in the ever-expanding field of nursing informatics, in school nursing which may or may not be physically demanding depending on the school, and other nonhospital nursing jobs. These nurses typically say that they could not do a hospital nursing job because of their physical disabilities. One nurse said

I've done a lot of working with IT (information technology) ... which I love and it takes pressure off my joints ... because it's a lot ... at my desk. ... I have a keyboard that is ergonomically correct. I have a mouse pad that is helpful ergonomically and those are the ways that I've compensated. ... I have a chair that's comfortable and I can adjust height and how I'm sitting. ... You learn to position yourself differently if something's uncomfortable but basically a lot of what I do is like an outpatient clinic versus an inpatient setting. I don't have to lift patients. I don't have to turn patients. I don't have to do a lot of physical stuff with my job which if I were in a hospital situation, I don't think I'd still be in nursing at this point. I'm almost positive I would not be. ... I'm working for the benefits right now and I feel pressured to keep this job ... so I can retire. ...

Another nurse with joint arthralgias and pain related to a motor vehicle accident described moving from hospital nursing to occupational health nursing to travel nursing in prisons. This nurse had trouble standing but in most of her travel assignments she was supervising.

> I usually did supervising. I was either the manager of the health services or I was director of nursing. In one or two sites, I had to be a staff nurse.... But at each job, I was able to get off my feet. When I was staff nursing for prisons, I had to do med pass so that meant standing at a window and the inmates would come and take their medications from me. That wasn't too bad because med pass would last half hour, forty-five minutes and then I could go back to the main office and sit down and do my paperwork.

She later worked in home care making home visits and eventually worked private duty. She then became a nurse consultant for a halfway house. Not all of her job transitions were precipitated by her disability but the disability played a significant role in the job choices she made. Before she left hospital work, she had tried to get administration to give her light duty.

> I said why don't you put me in cardiac care and I can sit in front of the monitors and then I can read the monitors and they just couldn't go there.... They just couldn't make the transition to something other than where I'd been before. They really didn't want me back until I could actually spend a day on my feet walking around the unit and it was my head nurse that was agreeable to let me work with a cane, but I could imagine other head nurses saying no, you have to be appliance free to come back.

She worked with a cane for a while but she had to rest one day for ever day she worked and she began to sense a change in the way others viewed her.

One nurse who was working at a community hospital was leaving after her shift one night and had a car accident. She was recovering from it for a long time and was left with a seizure disorder and the inability to walk unassisted. Thankfully, she was offered a job that primarily involved patient teaching. The job did not work out because, in her view, she was taken advantage of because of her disability. As a result, the nurse moved to another state and temporarily left nursing altogether. She tried to go back to nursing but was told that if she couldn't do CPR, then she could not practice on the floor. "I was always with other nurses. I was on the floors with other nurses and I kept saying 'Look, I can do everything else, I'm young, I'm gonna get my strength back. I'll work on [CPR]. I can do one hand.'"

This nurse later applied for a position in the intensive care unit (ICU) at a different hospital.

> They hired me for ICU ... and I had to do CPR and I practiced it and I learned to do it like this and it hurt like a son of a gun but

I did it and I passed, no problem, I did just fine. So, it was just a question of getting my arms stronger.... So I got hired for that... took extra courses. I started working for my bachelor's [degree].

However, she also ran into difficulty with this job. At this point, she was still limping from her accident despite the length of time that had passed and she still had many visible stitches along with an arm that was "locked" and could not bend.

I had to ask—they had to have a stool because we still just had 8 hour shifts but my ankles always had swelling.... And at first there was "We can't have people trip over a stool." I asked "Well then, could I have beds that are near the window so I can sit on the radiator?" At first, that was an issue but eventually got them to allow me to do that. I never considered myself handicapped. I never asked for a handicap sticker until the last couple of years. I'm giving in for one. But again, it was allowed. I always had to go through channels. I never made it difficult. I've always worked weekends, evenings. I think most people had no idea that I had a handicap at all.... Being a handicapped nurse was not an issue in my life much until the last 5 years really and now it's an enormous issue and one that I'm dealing with in a way that I'm not sure is going to help me help others; I'm just appalled and stunned [about] what's going on in my life right now as a handicapped person.

This nurse left the ICU because she moved and began working with troubled adolescents. "I just think, working with these screwed up kids, it's been a real place in my life, it's a highlight for me.... It's been a wonderful thing." She also pursued and obtained her master's degree in nursing. She was soon offered a job teaching at a school of nursing.

They got me a wonderfully comfortable chair because they knew I was handicapped. Not a question was asked. They asked "Are you okay? Do you need anything because of the handicap?" There were handicapped parking places and if I asked for anything because of my handicap, because they are a state institution, I believe I would have had it.

She later went on to practice as a nurse practitioner in an ambulatory care center.

A nurse with a neuromuscular disease was told to stop her current nursing job because of her limitations.

I talked to my physician because he had sent a letter to the director saying "I don't want her to do that and I don't want her to do this but she is capable of doing this and this and this" but they didn't care that I was capable of doing certain things; they were more concerned about the things I couldn't do than what I could do.

This is not at all uncommon among the nurses studied. Much emphasis is placed on their inability to perform certain functions while less, if any, time is spent determining what they can do and in what other ways their skills and abilities can be used in nursing. When this nurse was asked if anyone offered her an opportunity to do other types of nursing work, she responded:

No, no. . . . I was working in the operating room (OR) when I was first diagnosed and then I was shifted to the admissions area of that department. I had told the director . . . because they were having trouble getting nurses, I said "You need a course here for RNs who are interested in becoming OR nurses" and she said "Well, yeah, we do need that but we need to get the numbers up first." As a result, all of the nurses that they hired were taught by other nurses who had been taught by other nurses who were not OR nurses. [They] were taught . . . what you would do but there was no theory behind it; there was no why you do this this way. . . . I was the only certified nurse in the whole department and I had been trained to be a registered nurse OR assistant so I could suture, I could do other kinds of things. . . . There were so many other things that I could have done, but they weren't going to keep me.

She was taken out of the OR despite having been an OR nurse for 30 years and was asked to go to the ambulatory surgery unit to admit and discharge patients. In this case, the hospital made an effort to retain her by placing her in a different setting within the hospital.

I wouldn't be on call anymore and I wouldn't be subject to handling heavy trays of instruments. . . . I fought it at first because I didn't want to do it 'cause I know how busy that kind of place can be and I said I don't have that kind of energy to work there and they said "Why don't you just try it?" and I said okay in an effort to stay employed. I was willing to try anything to stay employed. Guess what? I started to love it even though it had a hectic pace. . . . I had one particular assistant there who bent over backwards to help me. . . . She was a nursing assistant; she wasn't even an LPN or RN.

When her physician wrote a letter to the hospital saying that she shouldn't work later hours or overtime "... they told me they were not going to create [a] position for me." This nurse never pursued any legal action and no longer pursued a job in nursing. "... I got involved in my church ... and I work on a committee where I go visit homebound parishioners." While she was not performing nursing care per se, she did visit people who were disabled themselves or chronically ill and her fellow committee members appreciated that she was visiting those people because of her nursing knowledge. She found volunteering rewarding and it helped fill the gap left by her grief over not being able to work in nursing.

Another nurse with disabling allergies and fibromyalgia was unable to continue her hospital work and moved into ICU care at home. "I'm taking care of an 18 month old on a ventilator. She's got a feeding tube. She's got pulmonary disease...." She had tried to get hospital ICU jobs but she did not have any luck.

> Because you have to float, you have to do nights. In one place I interviewed, [the administrator] said that in their ICU, they have to float out and also do their med-surg (medical surgical) floor. She said it is hard work for an ICU nurse to run up and down that floor. "They're 20 rooms long," she said, "but everybody has to do it and because you can't do it you're not going to be very much of a team player." That is why I didn't get that job.

Some nurses end up retiring early if it is an option, because they cannot find or get help to find a job that they can do in nursing. One public health nurse who taught in an academic setting but who also took nursing students to third world countries to provide care to underserved people found that she had to carefully think of what she wanted to do and could do.

> I could have taken eight students to the VNA (Visiting Nurse Association) and used the telephone to check [on how they were doing during the day], but I didn't. I wasn't interested in that type of job anymore ... and I think this is true of people who get into public health, they kind of have a sense of risk and adventure ... you probably know early enough that's why you get into public health. But at a certain point I had to look up and see what the balance was, so I plan my retirement.... I am trying to wind down.... I can see now, in retrospect, how I could have done things differently, but at the time you are just basically trying to get through every day.

Another nurse suffered a traumatic hearing loss and despite hearing aids did not feel that she should go back to nursing in case she couldn't hear the patients. She did not realize the severity of the hearing loss until she had an experience with a patient.

> I was on duty one night alone and the signal light was on and I did not hear it. I made continuous rounds. I went in and found the lady had had her signal light on. . . . When I got there, she was in distress and she said "I've had this on for a half an hour."

She had been working for an agency that employed nurses in various places and told the agency that she should no longer be given any patient assignments.

> After it sunk in that I was really more incapacitated than I realized. After I got my hearing aids, I tried [going back to work] again. That was before I finally decided not to and I just couldn't hear what people were [saying], especially females. Male voices, I . . . really don't have any problems with. . . . [The administrator] just wanted warm bodies, couldn't care less what their abilities were. . . . I said "I just don't think I can do that anymore, I just had this bad experience. . . . I can't trust my hearing."

When asked why she decided not to go back and take care of patients, she said "I was afraid of it." When asked if she had pursued other types of nursing she responded:

> I just miss doing something and I suppose I could do paperwork. I really don't know what's out there. But, you know, interestingly enough, a lot of very health-qualified educated nurses like to do that paperwork Monday through Friday. I just haven't looked. . . .

It often takes a change in mindset to gear oneself up to look for jobs in nursing that are very different from what the nurse had previously done or how they saw themselves as nurses. This is particularly difficult when the nurse does not receive any assistance in finding a job that might suit her or his abilities.

AN UNEXPECTED BENEFIT

Sometimes the move from one type of nursing to another or out of nursing, whether self-imposed or directed by others, turns out to be a good thing. Some nurses felt that because of the disability, they went on to higher education and moved into new fields of nursing. Others felt that leaving their jobs opened up new possibilities for them. It is interesting to note that many of the nurses eventually viewed the change in career or job as something positive. One nurse with post polio syndrome worked parttime visiting military families, many of whom included new mothers and babies. When asked if her disabilities influenced her career decisions she answered:

> I think disabilities and desires. I knew that with my disabilities that I could not work a straight 8-hour day plus, on my feet.... There's a creative part of me that was never developed and I really need to do that just for [me].... I had not been able to do that before and I really enjoyed it.

When asked if having a disability particularly one that developed in her adolescent years, had changed how she felt about nursing, she said that the disability had been an influence on her decision to go into nursing.

> Well, I felt that I had more empathy for people. I certainly knew what it felt like to be in pain, and have a lot of surgeries, and for physicians not to be honest.... I had a lot of problems with body image and self-esteem.... I had a lot of problems with kids at school, because I had so much surgery that I knew I couldn't do silly things because I could fall, break my arm, and have to go through things all over again.... I didn't get invited places.... It kept me from doing a lot of things that high school kids did....

One nurse expressed her satisfaction that she had work in nursing that she could do and which she loved:

> Economically, it would be a tough thing [not to be able to work] but luckily I found college health and it's really been a lifesaver for me in terms of career because I loved it to start with and then too it's been a job that I can do.

Another nurse with post polio syndrome realized that despite all of the jobs she had done she could no longer work full time and needed to find something that she could do that would use her nursing knowledge but that wouldn't completely drain her.

> Once a month I lead the [disability] support group and I was involved for several years at the state level also with [a] post polio group and I've done that. Then a couple of years ago I said.... I'm sure [there are] things I could do so I started working, volunteering for the Red Cross and in their blood collection center.

> I liked that better than going out in the community.... I could do it for 2 hours, that was about it. Running around helping people when I could still use my nursing. I could still do an assessment because I did assess people for whether or not they were reacting to having their blood taken or whatever.... Then I did some sitting down and just greeting people and that was nice.

This nurse later got involved in parish or congregational nursing: "I'm not using my nursing license. I'm not getting paid as a nurse but I am doing senior visiting... and it's going to one person's home.... I'm using my psych nursing skills and [all] kinds of nursing skills."

Another nurse had limitations in the function of one knee and was given a temporary desk job during which she worked on paperwork that needed to be done by the unit. The plan was for her to eventually go back to bedside care but she was needed in this sedentary desk job and continued to do it despite not having an official new position or title. While doing the job she came to enjoy the work.

> It's made me very strong in areas that I never imagined that I'd be strong in.... The administrative side of things, being responsible for delegation, education, things like that, was never something I imagined doing, let alone enjoying.

It is interesting that many nurses with disabilities who left their jobs to go back to school or who, as in this case, took other jobs came to enjoy them and found an unexplored area of themselves. This nurse decided to take these new skills and apply for an administrative job elsewhere in nursing.

> [Because of] my disability, I cannot provide bedside care. There's things that I still love about xxx [specialty of nursing] nursing, that I can do again away from the bedside and those are the things I want to focus on as I move forward with my education.

She said that she was leaving the institution she had worked for because she did not get any recognition for the work she did in her temporary job and didn't feel that her contributions as a nurse were recognized because of her disability.

> I know I can contribute in a completely different and new way and still be a member of the team and I'd like that opportunity to show that despite having this disability, I can still help you guys. I can still be really valuable on the floor.

One nurse who temporarily could not do bedside care because of surgery on her leg was given desk work so that she could complete several projects that the unit was required to complete. She had been told that she had one week to get back to full capacity and when she could not, she was allowed to work under her previous job description of bedside care while performing desk work. She had a hard time adjusting at first because the other nurses thought she was shown favoritism and because she had to struggle to get a computer and a phone to be able to do the work but as time went by, she realized that she liked the type of policy work that was involved and decided to pursue a degree in Human Services.

> I wasn't ever planning on going beyond my associate's [degree]. I had 4 years of college and was just a couple of credits shy of getting my bachelor's in nursing but because it ... wouldn't change the financial outcome, I didn't bother pursuing it but as of this coming [week] I graduate with my bachelor's ... [in] Human Services ... and then I'm starting the master's program in January ... again in Human Services with the idea that I may even pursue ... a doctorate in health care administration or something of that nature because it's something that I just really truly enjoy.... I never realized how much I could do for the patients away from the bedside.

MAKING A CHOICE AND GIVING IT A TRY

Taking a chance and trying something new is frequently the only way the nurse with a disability can find out whether or not to stay in nursing. The nurse with a disability has to seriously consider whether he or she can face yet another possible rejection or accept whatever position they can get in lieu of what they'd like to do. However, nurses must be realistic and self-aware regarding their own limitations and strengths before approaching something new in nursing. One nurse educator discussed her thought processes regarding staying in academe.

> I think the only thing about it is it's a very hectic fast paced environment if you're going to meet all of the expectations. I kind of gave up on some of the potential goals, like I gave up on making professor or publishing because I would have liked to. I gave up certain things so I could keep other things going. Some of that has been a personal choice, just so I could keep going. I think looking back on it there have been a significant number of semesters where I wasn't really very good at that, I didn't feel very good.

Another nurse who worked in intensive care felt that despite certain disabilities, a nurse should be able to continue in that setting.

> To me, a nurse [who] has got the qualities to work in an ICU should work in ICU. Sometimes, they can go into education and help but at the same time, they're still losing a lot of their skills if they're not using them. They could be a preceptor a little bit more frequently, they could do a lot of teaching other nurses.

An advanced practice nurse who used a wheelchair described changing jobs from one clinical practice to another as a result of her interactions with the physician who owned the practice.

> There was a job prior to this ... a private practice, it was a one-physician practice and a friend referred me to this position because I was a new nurse practitioner and he was a really good teacher, the physician who worked there, so it would be a good spot for me to kind of get some guidance. He made no qualms about saying that he didn't know if I could do the job because of my disability. He basically said I know I'm supposed to be equal opportunity and not supposed to hold your disability against you but you know this is the real world and these are my exam rooms and this is the space that I have and this is what we have to work with. So I basically had to convince him to give me a try. I said we're not gonna know whether or not you think I can do this until I show you, so all I'm asking is that you give me a shot and we'll see how it goes. He agreed to put me on some sort of probationary status for like a week or two where I could work there, see the patients. I knew I could do it. I just had to show him I could do it so ... this is just a trial run for him because he needs reassurance. I did what I always do and took care of patients perfectly well and he hired me quickly after that but that was a really difficult job. I ended up having to leave that job because the discrimination there was just awful.

This nurse practitioner said that the physician developed a nickname for her that was derogatory toward someone with a disability.

> I had to quit, I couldn't take it. It was awful. He would say it in front of patients, too, which was just so humiliating.

Another nurse who had severe arthritis moved from working in the emergency department to staffing the recovery room in a clinic that performed outpatient surgical procedures. She was isolated back in recovery and did not see other staff very much but felt that the work itself was manageable given her disabilities. When asked if she wanted to stay in nursing she responded:

> I would like to, very much, 'cause I love it. [The position I am in now is] so boring, it's nauseating. The day takes forever . . . but I'm just grateful for the job and I like the camaraderie with the staff that I'm working with so it makes it worthwhile. . . . I'm seeing people and it's getting me out of my house where I'm able to interact with people again. It's a change in nursing and I get some respect. . . . Just the fact that they call you nurse and they . . . acknowledge my experience, just made me feel better. . . . Instead of negatives, you get a positive.

A nurse said about nursing: "I miss in nursing . . . the working really fast. . . . You always have more to do in a short period of time. I certainly could do that but . . . I'm not as fast. . . . I'm not like what I used to be."

ACCEPTING THE LIMITATIONS

Often a nurse has to make the decision to leave the job or nursing altogether. At such times, the nurse tries to accept the fact and find a way to justify the change in careers. Some choose a specific area of nursing for a reason. Other times, the area of nursing chooses them because their choices are limited due to the disability. As one nurse said: "If I were in another field of nursing it would make a big difference because . . . I could [not] stand on my feet for 8 hours. There is no way in the world I could do that."

Sometimes, a nurse with a disability has to open him or herself up to opportunities in nursing they never previously thought they'd pursue. One nurse described this experience: ". . . When I was in nursing school and I did my rotation, I actually liked school nursing but why I am doing it now is mostly—I'm gonna say 95% of it is because of my disability. . . ."

Older nurses who have retired from more physically demanding jobs may also choose jobs that are still in nursing but are manageable despite their age-associated disabilities. School nursing is one such job option, depending on the type and size of the school.

> Most of the school nurses have retired from working in a hospital and they wanna still do nursing but they don't want to work as a hospital nurse so it's much more pleasant than working in a hospital. . . . So I chose this because I like kids and I like nursing.

Another nurse who had had cancer and had an ostomy as a result moved into a desk job giving advice to patients over the phone:

> Well I must say that the reason I was actually looking for this job was that I had had shoulder surgery. . . . I was looking for a job that was less physically taxing and that's how I fell into this job.

When asked if there were any nursing jobs she felt she could not do at this point, she responded:

> I would say that heavy lifting would be out completely. I would say OR (operating room) is out . . . any kind of prolonged clinical activity would be out, bedside nursing would be out.

One nurse has three jobs that mostly involve teaching and computer work. She was able to change from clinical teaching with students to classroom teaching.

> I've been able to kind of segue from the clinical aspect where I'm on my feet for a long period of time to being in the classroom where I can go up and down and ask people to help me when needed: lifting help and whatnot. I was able to choose what I wanted to do and, yes, I made that choice because obviously it's much easier physically for me to do that. I worked as a home care nurse for almost 20 years, most of that time I worked full time or at least four full days a week, which required me seeing usually an average of six patients a day, a lot for them total care so I had to turn and lift and position patients to do my care as well as carrying supplies in and out of houses and going up three flights of stairs and whatever it entailed for me to get to the patient and do my job. About the time when I was diagnosed and I was feeling so fatigued and having the pain, I was trying to find ways to alter the way I did my job to accommodate my disability and then . . . someone called about the teaching position and I thought—I always loved teaching, maybe that'll be a bit easier . . . because I found I couldn't do what I was expected to do anymore.

This nurse stayed in home care along with taking the teaching position but she switched to another agency that allowed her to work on a per-visit basis instead of full time.

> I switched over because I really didn't want to give up seeing clients so this is a per-visit position as opposed to working full

time and they needed someone and it just happened that that was a good place for me to go and they call me when they need me. . . . [It's] sort of at will and it works out better for me.

She had asked the first home health agency to allow her to work less than full time and they refused.

Actually, I originally asked them if I could go down to working 2 days a week because I couldn't do the full 4 days doing all that heavy work . . . and they said, no, that I could stay full time or I could not be there, so I immediately went and got a job someplace else, being per visit. . . . They knew [I had a disability] because I had had several surgeries and they knew I had back issues though I didn't have the arthritis diagnosis yet. . . . I found that I really like the teaching so now I've changed over to that in my career plans but everyone I work with is very helpful and supportive. It's a good group. . . . [Regarding the home care position] I am in a position to choose.

In her part-time home care position, she can choose which patients she is willing to see. When she is called to make a visit, she asks if the patient requires total care, lifting, moving or other physical work on her part. If so, she does not take that patient. If she arrives at a patient's home and finds that the patient requires physical care, she will not leave the patient but does her best to provide the care even if she has to compensate or move more slowly.

In her teaching role, this nurse has found ways to compensate for what she cannot easily do because of her disabilities:

I find the tallest student and say you're my helper . . . climb up and get things. I have the strong students carry things for me . . . and they're all very willing to help. . . . When I'm working in the clinical skills lab if we have to work with the manikins I have someone move them and I just ask people to do it now instead of trying to do it myself.

A nurse with a hearing impairment described how she took her current job as a school nurse and health counselor because it enabled her to be closer to an ill family member and care for them during her breaks, but that she was considering whether her disabilities now warranted another career change.

I'm starting to say maybe I should look for something else or should I file [for] disability. . . . I've always worked all my life and

> I do get depressed. I'll tell you it does depress me and I went to the Bureau of Rehab. That's how I got these hearing aids actually.... [They] pay for your hearing aids because they're very expensive and your insurance doesn't cover them.

When this nurse considers a career change she thinks of going into social work "where I'm close to the person to communicate [and] I could hear better like one-on-one." This nurse is fortunate to have a degree in addition to her nursing degree that gives her the option of going into social work. She went back to school for the non-nursing degree because of her disability so she would "not have to be in a critical situation where someone's giving orders to do something and I didn't comprehend exactly what they said."

Having a chronic illness or disability can induce feelings of depression especially when the nurse is limited in the work she can do. A nurse with rheumatoid arthritis said that she made a career change to a desk job because of her disability.

> For me it's been not so much going in with a set disability as it has been a progression. I've had changes in my joints from the rheumatoid [arthritis], the associated problems that go with it, dealing with depression, just dealing with fatigue issues, like less mobility.... So what I've found is just a growing inability to be on my feet, to work longer shifts, to do the physical aspects of caring for patients and that's kind of what moved me into more of a desk type of position.... I had been working in a similar position in a local hospital and I left there to do some consulting which required some degree of travel and then I had to go off work for about 6 months and I just knew I couldn't physically handle the travel at this point so this position was really good because it doesn't require travel. I completely work from home and so that was a large part of my decision for this particular position.

This nurse had been working in a cardiac unit, which required a lot of physical activity, prior to her diagnosis. She continued to do that for several years after her diagnosis. She explained that because her diseases were exacerbated by stress, she needed to use her sick time and vacation time to take days off for stress relief. This did no leave her any time for actual vacations. She moved into a job as a database coordinator. Her immediate manager also had a chronic disease and was consequently very supportive of this nurse. However, "the supervisors at the next level up really didn't understand and some of my coworkers made things kind of difficult...."

> It came to a point. . . . I wasn't fired per se, they didn't do away with my position; they kind of restructured my position and so at that time they offered me a severance and the way they worked [it] was you got paid for a month and during that time you could reapply for other positions within the institution and if you found something you wanted, it wasn't quite handled like a transfer. If you get to the end of that month [and you hadn't found something else] then [it would be] as if you resigned. . . . And what I found when that happened is that honestly I had probably stayed too long. . . . I just recognized I couldn't do it at all and honestly what I should've done at that point was just requested they let me go out on disability at that time as opposed to doing the agreement where I just left and at that time I planned on applying for other positions but I knew I couldn't handle anything with a higher degree of physicality. There just wasn't anything I felt like I could apply for and within a matter of weeks I realized that I probably couldn't go back to anything along those lines at that time.

This nurse had to educate the upper management about compliance with ADA and medical leave but began to feel that her job was in jeopardy about a year or so before she left the job. Fortunately, she had a family member who was well versed in disability laws and rights so she was able to talk with Human Resources department at work about what she needed.

> I didn't need a lot of physical accommodations at the time. It was . . . before they were really conscious of a lot of ergonomic type of evaluations, but what I needed was having days I couldn't work to full capacity or where I had to miss days and [be on] medical leave. Once [upper management] were educated along those lines, they were good about providing it. . . .

Eventually this nurse did feel forced out of this job but she sought and acquired a position in nurse informatics, teaching nurses about electronic records and helping health care providers to comply with new guidelines. The job has turned out to be ideal for her given her disability.

> I'm able to pretty much sit all day, get up, take breaks when I need to. Honestly, where I'm at with my RA right now, working from home is ideal. I think even the stress of even getting up and going to an office would probably be enough that I don't even think I'd be able to work at this point.

In this job, she is provided with the accommodations she needs and people are supportive because of what she brings to the table.

> They were very open to getting what I needed as far as the work station. I actually work with people who are much more understanding of the issues, very willing to let me take the time I needed.... I still have the issues of ... driving myself harder than I should....

Another nurse spoke of her emotions when she realized that because she was in pain, she would have to change the way she thought about nursing.

> [In] undergraduate nursing education, they tell you that there's these opportunities but you don't think about it, you're just thinking about being at the bedside passing pills and looking at lab work and I just never dreamed that [administration] would ever be anything I was interested in and then when I started realizing "Oh my.... I'm in pain constantly. I can't be at the bedside. What am I going to do. I'm not gonna be able to be a nurse anymore" and then it was like ... a light bulb! ... There are things in nursing that I can do that aren't at the bedside.

In this case the nurse decided not to leave nursing but did leave the bedside for administration. She also decided to pursue higher education. While recovering from surgery, this nurse was given a sedentary job in which she was behind a desk. She did not feel supported despite the transition to light duty.

> They weren't that helpful. At first, I still think they were ... jealous is a strong word, but I think that they really looked at me like why is she still here? She's not performing. She's not being a nurse so why is she still here? Especially, when I didn't have to come in on the weekends anymore and I didn't have to work holidays anymore....

Sometimes a nurse happens to already be working in a job that turns out to be the best job for them once they become disabled.

A nurse anesthetist commented:

> Of all the fields of nursing that I could've picked, for whatever reason the plans lined up and I made the best possible choice of being able to be active in nursing with minimal physical demands.

Life would've been much harder if I had chosen to be a floor nurse or an ER nurse on my feet constantly for 8 to 10 hours. It would've been much more difficult had I been in those roles.

This nurse went into nurse anesthesia because of his experience as a child with a chronic, painful illness.

Quite honestly, I went into anesthesia as sublimation. . . . As a kid . . . and you ask for pain medicine I was literally told by nursing personnel, "John Wayne doesn't use pain medicine, why do you?" . . . I've spent the rest of my life trying to sublimate and take pain away for other people.

If nurses with disabilities are aware or made aware of job opportunities that will allow them to remain in nursing, they are likely to stay in nursing because they love what they do and they want to continue to help others. Even when they are eligible to retire or to get disability benefits they may choose not to because they want to continue to work as nurses. One nurse who is an educator in an academic setting decided to keep working after she suffered an injury that caused her to be disabled because she loves to teach.

I could've retired. I could've taken the disability benefits beyond what I had already used but I really wanted to go back to teaching and so I just decided that I would and see how it went . . . I know my limitations. I know what kinds of things I need to accommodate myself to or acclimate myself to and that's made a difference. I don't feel quite as awkward and uncomfortable as I used to. . . .

SOLUTIONS

Chapter 8 will discuss possible solutions in detail. It is worthwhile to keep in mind that given the choice, nurses with disabilities do seem to want to continue to work as nurses. Nurse leaders and administrators can capitalize on this desire to keep working by making it possible for nurses with disabilities to work.

Options within each individual organization will vary depending on the type and scope of the organization. However, it is up to nurse leaders to keep an open mind about the nurse with a disability, to look beyond the disability to what matters: nursing knowledge, expertise, motivation, enthusiasm, readiness to learn, and willingness to work. Nurse leaders should consider the work that needs to be done and how it might be reconfigured to make the most of the individual nurse's skills and abilities rather than emphasizing whether or not they can walk, run, or lift patients. Every job has its own requirements but how many of those so-called requirements are truly necessary to doing the job effectively. In patient care, the quality of the care is the ultimate indicator of nursing excellence. The question is whether patients can receive better care from a knowledgeable nurse who may need assistance with mobility or from a physically able nurse who does not have high level of knowledge or the ability to think critically or quickly in a crisis situation.

There are many nursing jobs that do not involve direct patient care. In those cases (with some exceptions), it is difficult to understand why a nurse with a physical and/or sensory disability could not perform them well. So far, this book has raised some examples in which nurses with disabilities have successfully transitioned from one nursing job to another despite having a disability. Among them are the nurse educator role, nurse informatics, desk work, some types of home care, consultation, and some types of advanced practice nursing. There are undoubtedly others. However, these examples illustrate that it *can* be done and moreover that it *should* be done so we don't lose valuable nurses to the profession.

REFERENCE

Neal-Boylan, L. J. (2012). An exploration and comparison of the worklife experiences of registered nurses and physicians with permanent physical and/or sensory disabilities. *Rehabilitation Nursing, 37*(1), 3–10.

5

Does Having a Disability Compromise Patient Safety?

Andrew, a 55-year-old registered nurse, had a left, below-the-knee amputation as a result of a motor vehicle accident. He had worked in the emergency department (ED) of a community hospital for the past 10 years. Initially, he came back to work using crutches and his manager put him behind the triage desk so he wouldn't have to walk too much, but eventually he was fitted for a prosthetic leg and felt that he could move almost as well as he did before. His colleagues and manager had been supportive during his long convalescence and his return to work but when he obtained his prosthesis and declared that he was ready to resume caring for patients in the ED, he was told that his inability to move quickly might jeopardize patient safety. Andrew was able to demonstrate that he could move almost as quickly as the other nurses, albeit with a limp but that did not seem to satisfy everyone. A special staff meeting was held in which the staff was encouraged to discuss whether they felt that Andrew could keep up sufficiently to manage patients on his own. During this meeting, Andrew felt very much singled out and was the recipient of comments, that while sympathetic, clearly demonstrated a loss of confidence in Andrew's ability to provide safe patient care. Despite his best efforts, Andrew was unable to overcome this perception. He found work in an ED at another hospital and made sure not to reveal that he had a prosthetic leg. Everyone seemed satisfied with his performance.

Regard for patient safety is often the reason why nurses with disabilities leave their jobs. They may fear that they will jeopardize patient safety and/or others may feel that the nurse will jeopardize patient safety and, subsequently, push them out of the job. Interestingly, this was also a concern when the work lives of physicians and nurses with disabilities were compared. Physicians and those that employ them verbalized concern about the consequences of having a disability on patient safety (Neal-Boylan, 2012; Neal-Boylan, et al., 2012). Physicians and nurses are in the business of caring for others. It makes sense that they would put patient safety first. The problem arises when others assume that their disability will somehow prevent them from providing safe care. This chapter discusses the issue of patient safety with regard to nurses with disabilities from several perspectives. The voices of nurse recruiters, nurses with disabilities, and patients will be expressed and their points of view will be analyzed.

AN EXCUSE TO PUSH THE NURSE OUT

Interestingly, to date there have been no documented cases of patient injury that were directly caused by a nurse with a disability. Yet, it is testimony to the priority nurses place on the care of their patients that they should even consider leaving their jobs and sometimes nursing altogether because their disability might jeopardize patient safety. It doesn't appear that colleagues or administrators attempt to dissuade nurses with disabilities of the concern over patient safety. Instead, they seem to use this concern as a valid reason to discourage nurses from staying in their jobs. From the perspective of nurses with disabilities, this sometimes results from the need to find an excuse to push out a nurse who may not otherwise be performing as they'd like them to perform or who is not liked, or it may arise from ignorance or a lack of awareness of how a nurse with a disability might be able to compensate and perform safely. Many nurses with disabilities describe the apparent jealousy by others when the nurse with the disability is given accommodations such as shorter shifts or day shifts or is allowed to use compensatory techniques to practice.

Ignorance and lack of awareness, however, are poor excuses. Nurses care for people with chronic illnesses and acute or chronic disability as a matter of course in their everyday work. Most often patients arrive at health care facilities because they have had a temporary or permanent injury or illness. Illness can cause weakness, fatigue, reduced stamina, the need to use assistive devices to aid mobility or to use the assistance of another person to ambulate or perform activities of daily living. To these patients, nurses typically show concern and compassion while educating others to treat them just as they would anyone else.

NURSES DON'T CARE FOR EACH OTHER

Nurses are trained to care for those who cannot care for themselves. Yet, according to many nurses with disabilities, their colleagues do not tend to show the same awareness or compassion for nurses who are ill or disabled. Perhaps this derives from working in high pressure environments with never enough staff and tremendous responsibility. The overriding concern of the nurse may be to protect him- or herself and when someone else cannot pull their own weight there is a need for those who are fully able bodied to pick up the slack. This means that the other staff often work harder or longer or do things that they would prefer not to do. It is not unreasonable for nurses to feel weighed down by having to compensate for what another nurse cannot do. The interesting thing, however, is that many of the nurses with disabilities say that they can do their work if they are allowed to make compensations or if they are enabled and encouraged to work in nursing jobs that do not require them to compensate.

NURSES WITH DISABILITIES RECOGNIZE THEIR LIMITATIONS

Many nurses with disabilities acknowledge that they may not be able to work in every type of nursing setting, depending on their disability. They acknowledge that certain abilities are required to perform safe patient care. However, it appears to them that there is little opportunity for an in-between solution. In other words, for many, it is a question of whether or not they can continue to do the job they have been doing in the exact way it has always been done. The alternative is that they leave nursing. Some go back to school, others engage in volunteer work and use their nursing skills, but it appears that many would stay in nursing as RNs if they were offered or made aware of opportunities in which they could use their expertise despite the disability.

THE HEARING-IMPAIRED NURSE

Difficulty hearing seems to be a disability that is on the rise among nurses. One study found that of the nurse participants who came from a variety of work settings, the nurses with trouble hearing who worked in hospital settings were more at risk of leaving their jobs than were nurses with hearing problems who worked in other settings. This may be related to working in a hospital setting and not necessarily to having a hearing problem. However, nurses with hearing disabilities who were interviewed described their frustration working in hospital settings. In a study of nurses with sensory disabilities, the length of time one had spent working as a nurse was associated with trouble hearing even though age was not (Neal-Boylan, Fennie, & Baldauf-Wagner, 2011). This same study found that nurses who had some or severe difficulty with sensory function were no longer working in nursing. This validated work from previous studies that found that nurses with disabilities tend to leave nursing.

One nurse recruiter described a labor and delivery nurse with deafness who worked at her facility.

> Now we could accommodate by [putting devices on] all the phones and so forth but it was interesting, many of the physicians refused to work with her. They were afraid that they would say something in terms of instructions . . . in the labor room and turn to her and say "get me this, get me that" and she wouldn't be able to hear them. So, it became a huge issue. They felt like her limitation could actually influence patient safety . . . but you could see how that could extend itself to a nurse who was less mobile, if [what was needed was] time sensitive, if the thing the physician was requesting or the things the patient needed were time sensitive.

Another nurse manager in critical care commented about how an inability to hear well might jeopardize patient safety.

> You're expected to answer your own alarms. . . . So, I think in critical care . . . that would be pretty essential. . . . You know there are a number of things which you have to be able to do with your senses to be in critical care. . . . There are impairments that would [not be suitable] because of the safety of the patients. . . . I think nurses with hearing disabilities . . . could work in the less alarm driven environments.

Is it possible by just paying very close attention to the monitors for the nurse to be aware of developments without actually hearing the alarms? As technology advances, there will likely be alternatives to alarms or additional signs to warn nurses of problems patients are having that might enable a nurse with a hearing disability to work in critical care.

A nurse with hearing loss felt that there are many jobs which she would be unsafe performing.

> I wouldn't want to be working on an intensive care unit. I wouldn't want to be working in anything requiring all of your senses or even alone. . . . Another thing, asking people to repeat. [The] patient doesn't feel like repeating. . . . Asking people "What did you say? What was it you wanted?" Or . . . when you don't hear right, you respond by what you think you heard, so when you do something different . . . it's a perceptive disability. You can do your best to meet what people are asking for but sometimes it's called faking it. . . . If [people] turn their backs to me and I don't always wear

> these [hearing aids] and I think they said . . . this and then it turns out, oh no, I am doing something different . . . I just can't trust it.

Another nurse who lost her hearing suddenly left nursing because she realized that she could not hear patient alarm bells. She could not trust her hearing and felt that as much as it grieved her to leave her job, that patient safety was paramount. She voluntarily left bedside care but felt that her hearing disability should not prevent her from doing something else in nursing.

> I appreciate that they need people who have all their senses. . . . I think they have very legitimate needs. they want healthy people, they want reliable people. There must be something [I could do]. I just don't know. You can hire certified nursing assistants today to do a lot of what nurses used to do so I don't want to [do] less than what I'm qualified to do but it seems like some of my experiences and education [should count for something].

THE VISUALLY IMPAIRED NURSE

As nurses age, the normal process of aging often affects their ability to see as well as hear. Glasses typically correct the problem but sometimes a visual impairment can progress to be a disability. In the research study described earlier, a nurse with difficulty seeing described having to work harder than others to do what everyone else took for granted, namely reading and writing (Neal-Boylan et al., 2011). A nurse manager talked of trying very hard to accommodate a nurse with a visual impairment for as long as possible.

> Well, I had a nurse once that was going blind from her diabetes [and] that certainly was an issue for quite a long time. That's just an issue anyway, now, because the nurses are all old . . . and those little medication administration record squares were written for 20 year olds. I mean, I can't see them, so we just got magnifying things and kept her going as long as we could until she called it quits. . . . She ended up on nights 'cause there was less to do and she could take more time to do it . . . we just kept adjusting to try to accommodate her, but then she's just too blind, I mean there comes a point where you just can't be the nurse and be blind, you just can't.

Is there a place for the nurse who is blind? Can the experience and the expertise of the nurse be used on a patient advice line, for example?

In addition, perhaps there are settings in which Braille might be used for the nurse so information could be easily read. Advice lines, poison control centers, and insurance companies are among the settings in which Braille could be used to enable the blind nurse to read the information she or he needs to help the patient or caller. As technology advances, perhaps there will be others. A nurse who is not blind but who is visually impaired may only need larger print to be able to do his or her work effectively. To dismiss the nurse with a visual disability out of hand as not being able to work in nursing is unnecessary and unfair and wastes the nurse's accumulated knowledge. Particularly as nurses age and remain employed, it is unrealistic, not to mention discriminatory, to discard those nurses who do have experience and expertise merely because their ability to function physically or to hear or see has changed.

THE NURSE WHO IS OBESE

Interestingly, both nurse managers and nurses sometimes consider obesity to be a disability. One nurse manager discussed working with an obese nurse whom she felt jeopardized patient safety.

> I tried working with her . . . as far as . . . talking to her about her weight and the need to get that down and the need to go back to the doctor . . . and either she couldn't or wouldn't but anyway, she didn't, and in the end, I had to let her go, you know, because I didn't feel that she was safe on the floor.

The question arises as to whether it is an invasion of the privacy of the nurse or whether it is professionally appropriate for a nurse manager to suggest that the nurse lose weight or see her doctor. The nurse who was obese had trouble getting up off the floor and the manager worried that if a patient fell, that the nurse would not be able to assist the patient to get up. What about the other people on the floor or unit? If this nurse could not assist the patient by herself couldn't someone else assist her or the patient? This manager described another nurse with whom she worked who had cancer and resulting lymphedema.

> We tried to accommodate her as long as she could. Sometimes, I wondered how [with the lymphedema and wearing a compression sleeve] she was washing her hands or how she was wearing gloves, but there was always another nurse in the building and so that's why we tried to accommodate her there, [but] she couldn't do catheter insertion or something like that really, infection

control-wise anyway. So, the other nurse would do that. We let her work as long as we could until she started questioning her own judgment. It was starting to get into her brain, I think.

When asked how the nurse responded to being let go, the nurse manager answered "She understood. She really was coming around to that herself. She just didn't want to give it up. I mean, who does?" By "it" she said she meant independence. The nurse herself recognized that the changes in her cognition were affecting or could affect her ability to care for patients safely and she was willing to leave her position to protect her patients.

It is interesting to note that this same nurse manager did not feel that she could compensate for the obese nurse by having someone else assist her if a patient fell but did feel that she could accommodate the nurse with cancer, and for so long that the latter developed cognitive deficits from her illness. Is this an example of a value judgment of a person who has limited ability because she is obese versus a nurse who has cancer? Anyone who is able bodied and has strength, presumably, can assist in lifting a patient off of the floor. However, a registered nurse is needed to perform a catherization and must be very cautious about maintaining strict infection control. It appears that the obese nurse is not worth accommodating, perhaps because her disability may be self-induced. How do we know that that is the case and even if it is the case, do we, as nurses, opt not to care for patients who are obese even if they have caused their own obesity? Does the nurse who is obese lose his or her ability to think clearly and critically? The nurse with cancer did lose her ability to think clearly but it wasn't until she questioned her own ability to think clearly and her own judgment that it was acknowledged that she should no longer work.

THE NURSE WITH PAIN

One manager discussed under what conditions a nurse might not be safe if she or he had a disability: "... If you've got a lot of pain, you can't take a lot of pain medication, make the right decisions. Sometimes, we have to tell people to stay home when they are taking pain medications." One nurse with disabilities who took pain medication for her arthritis contacted the board of nursing in her state to find out if taking the medications would preclude her from working and whether she was required to tell her employer that she took the pain medication. She was told that it was only a matter of concern if her employers felt that she was unsafe. It makes sense that taking narcotic pain medications might jeopardize a nurse's ability to practice safely. However, it need not always be the case. The type, amount, and duration of the time the nurse has been taking the medication all impact the ability to function safely and effectively. This has to be determined on an individual basis.

FAIRNESS

Should accommodating a nurse with a disability be viewed as unfair to other nurses? The answer should be no. Is assuming that a nurse with a disability is unsafe fair to the nurse with a disability? Again, the answer should be no. Interestingly, one nurse manager described a nurse with musculoskeletal disabilities who the manager was anxious to keep. This nurse had sharp clinical skills and nursing experience but had also had a problem with her attendance.

> We haven't addressed that with her as much as we would have with somebody else.... We've tried to accommodate her situation . . . it's probably not fair, but we'd like to keep her because she is good in so many other ways. So, I guess in a way, that's accommodating her disability.

In this case, it seems that because the nurse is liked and has sharp clinical skills and experience, she is worth keeping and accommodating. The manager verbalized her worry that that was not fair to other nurses. This seems paradoxical. She seems to be saying that it is unfair to accommodate a nurse with a disability who is good at her job but who has a problem with attendance. However, it would seem to make more sense to accommodate the nurse who has a disability and then allow him or her to be measured using the same standards by which other nurses are measured, namely, the quality of their care.

ABILITY TO PRACTICE SAFELY

In many facilities and health care organizations, nurses must take and pass a physical examination in order to be hired. A nurse manager who worked in home care discussed the need for nurses with disabilities to be honest regarding their limitations and to pass the physical examination required of all nurses applying to work at the agency. She explained that her agency would be as accommodating as possible as long as the nurse would not jeopardize patient safety.

> If it's impacting patient care, for example [the nurse is] overmedicated or [has] psychological issues that [are] impacting patient care and maybe that's something that I need to bring up to HR [Human Resources] of what we could do about it.... When it comes to physical disabilities, we can accommodate those, but when it comes to patient care and their safety at home and rendering [care] safely, that would be something that we need to question.

Why should we question the ability of a nurse with disabilities to practice safely any more than we should question the ability of any nurse to practice safely? A nurse might come into work just having had a fight with his or her partner, angry and upset. This nurse's judgment might not be as clear as it might otherwise be. Another nurse might have a cold and feel ill and is likely to spread germs to her patients. Still another nurse might have only marginally passed his classes in nursing school and might be unsafe simply because he is not as bright as we would like him to be when having responsibility for patient care. Why, because a nurse has a physical impairment, do we seem to have a natural right to question his or her ability to practice safely more than we might question this ability in others?

Sometimes, in addition to a physical examination, nurses must undergo evaluation by a physical therapist to determine if they can handle the physical aspects of the job. One nurse manager commented. "They demonstrate the hands on with the physical therapist. They actually have to demonstrate that ability." This manager is committed to the idea that nurses with mobility issues would have difficulty providing safe patient care.

> There's lots of really important RN jobs ... that definitely impact the care around the patients that require possibly the physical piece that somebody without a limb or in a wheelchair or something is gonna have to demonstrate.

However, this manager also acknowledged that a nurse with a disability might be of value performing other nursing jobs.

> ... obviously my job, you know a nurse manager job, a case manager job, discharge planner, a utilization review, any of those things that I think ... obviously have a very valuable impact on the outcome of the patient but it's just that little bit further removed from the bedside hands on piece....

Patient safety is considered an issue if a nurse cannot respond quickly to emergencies and this naturally includes nurses who have trouble walking or walking quickly. When asked if there were specific criteria that would affect the ability of a nurse to work on their unit, one nurse manager responded:

> Well, clearly if somebody was not able to respond to a code situation . . . 'cause disabilities could be from anything, I'm thinking physical, you know, from a limp to not being able to walk. I couldn't say. First thing that comes to mind is patient safety. If it was something that was clearly going to prevent a care provider [from providing] safe patient care to a patient, we have to consider whether or not that person would qualify for that job.

When reading this, one is inclined to refer back to Chapter 2 which discusses why nurses with disabilities are leaving nursing. It seems that nurses who have visible physical disabilities may be prejudged when they go to interview for a position because managers and recruiters assume that they cannot provide safe patient care but don't seem to consider whether they might make another place for the nurse who may have value to the organization. This manager went on to elaborate using specific examples regarding when a nurse with a physical disability would jeopardize patient safety.

> Well, I guess I have to think of a person who needs to respond quickly, I mean in an acute care setting, say in a special care area, for example, or a critical care area or any area. . . . If . . . that person can demonstrate that their disability doesn't get in the way of [responding quickly] and . . . work is equal to the person without the disability then that would not have an impact on that patient's care.

This manager, in essence, is requiring the nurse to perform equally with nurses without disabilities. Is that necessary or just? What do we mean by "equally?" Perhaps the nurse with a disability cannot run or walk as quickly as a nurse without a disability, but has anyone compared the intellect of the two nurses or their abilities to make decisions or think critically? Are those measures of equality more important, ultimately, to patient safety than are physical standards, particularly when someone else might be physically able to perform those functions that do not require brain power?

OPTIONS

It might be possible to have certain nurses who are designated to respond to emergency situations and others who have other responsibilities that do not require running down a hallway or lifting a patient. What about the nurse who worked in acute care or critical care for many years and has the expertise that comes from experience? Could that nurse be used to monitor telemetry, give classes to other nurses, do most of the precepting of new nurses and student nurses, perform chart review, and perform many other tasks that do not require physical strength but do require expertise in that area of nursing? Perhaps a nurse with physical disabilities that prevents him or her from being able to respond to emergencies and is new to the organization might be assisted to find a position in another area of nursing that allows that nurse to make the best use of his or her abilities and allows that nurse to grow as a professional. One nurse manager who also had physical limitations of her own spoke specifically to this issue.

> At some point in the whole realm of nursing it would be nice to have something presented as far as options aside from clinical nursing. . . . There's a great nursing shortage but there's also a need for nurses in a lot of other areas and I just don't know that it seems to focus on clinical and . . . it would be nice to be able to just dabble [in] some of these other areas just to . . . get a taste for what's out there either down the road [when we are] older or if something does happen you don't feel that you are totally lost. . . . At least you know there's something there you could fall back on and maybe it's [not] so devastating.

There are so many different areas of nursing and probably many others yet to be explored as potential venues for nursing work. More and more, nursing students are exposed to different settings in which nurses practice simply as a response to the shortage of clinical placements in hospital settings. This exposure may have a positive impact on future nurses who may come to learn about and enjoy working in nonhospital settings. School nursing might be a reasonable option for some nurses with disabilities.

A school nurse described being in the position of having to respond to an emergency.

> I've never been in a position where I had to lift up a child. If a child is flat on the floor, you check to make sure the child is breathing and they're not injured and you call 911 and you call the parents and you get in touch with the principal. . . . I was in one school and I was in training where I had to climb up stairs to the second floor, that took me a bit longer but nobody's ever said anything . . . because the person you report to is the superintendent. . . . If there was an emergency, usually I'll go and maybe if the teacher would be there to help or they would call the janitor or . . . whoever they

call, but I've never [been] in a situation where I had to say no, I can't do this, I'm disabled.

This nurse found that school nursing was much more accommodating than were some other types of nursing and did not feel that anyone she worked with thought she was a threat to student safety. In the school environment, she found others who could help with the physical aspects of emergency care while she directed what needed to be done. She went into school nursing because she liked it but admitted that she had concerns about working in a hospital with her disability.

> I've had a [school] superintendent ask me why I wasn't working in a hospital and I told them because my foot was crushed and there was repair and I don't feel strong enough because you have to lift patients all day long and I was worried about hurting them and that's all [the school administration] said. They never questioned anything about it.

Perhaps, depending on the size of the school and the nature of the disability, a nurse with a disability who could not work in a hospital might be able to work productively and effectively in school nursing. Many nurses who have retired from hospital jobs seek positions as school nurses. Another school nurse was also clear that she didn't think having a disability compromised student safety:

> Other than doing CPR, getting on the ground and having to get back up again, the only situation that would come into play ... would be if two or three kids were down at one time, then I'd have to force myself up or call or do something to get over there. That would be the only situation [that might affect the safety of the students]. You are like the one nurse that's in charge of anyone that's in the school, teachers, anybody that walks into that building, you don't have enough nurses. They need at least two nurses where they only have one.

This nurse did describe a situation that might cause difficulty for some school nurses:

> Some schools, if the nurse is out you gotta get in your car and drive to another school to administer medication or take care of a serous situation. That's where that comes into play, that's where that's a problem, 'cause I'd have to do that too. It's not like I can run out of the building ... jump in my car real quickly. I have to walk out

of that building, walk as fast as I can, jump in my car, and get to the other school . . . that's going to take me twice as long.

To be sure she would not be in a position of jeopardizing a student's safety because of her slow mobility, this school nurse took advance precautions.

So it's a combination of having a disability and knowing if you're the nurse with the disability that you have to be able to maneuver yourself fast enough and it's usually within the same [school] district. So what I've done is ride around to the different schools and check out the situation before I applied for the job. Because I have to know that I have to be able to get in that building, see where I [would] park, and get over there fast enough. . . .

A nurse practitioner in a wheelchair said that when she interviewed for her job in a private practice there was discussion about what kinds of accommodations she would need but it was assumed that she could not respond quickly in an emergency.

When I applied for the job, there . . . was obviously discussion about, it wasn't really about the responsibilities. I think there was no doubt that I'd be able to fulfill the responsibilities. I think that . . . it just made sense that I wouldn't be the one to, you know, come to a code. . . . We didn't really actively discuss it but it's kind of, no, obviously I'm not going to be the one to run when there's a code called.

This nurse practitioner was valued for her expertise and it was assumed that she could not respond quickly in an emergency so other plans were put in place if an emergency were to occur. Could this be possible for nurses with disabilities who work in hospital settings?

A nurse manager expressed her concern about nurse educators with disabilities taking nursing students to the hospital for clinical practica.

I didn't put them in the clinical setting. . . . It was clear to me—this happened to be sending someone to a setting with children—and it was so difficult for this person or any person with a similar problem to physically engage in managing children in the setting. So for me it was kind of a no-brainer. I just decided well, this person could not go to that clinical setting or any clinical setting any longer so I used her in the classroom instead.

When asked if her concern involved patient safety, she replied:

> It was definitely safety. It was a safety issue for patients. It was a problem where I didn't believe the instructor would be able to do physically what was necessary to show the students how to physically work with these pediatric clients, lifting, moving, walking, whatever the kinds of things you need to do with kids, lifting kids primarily. So that was really my issue. It was a safety issue and it was also an educational issue for the students because I thought it was important. You can always have someone else lift and do but when you are working one on eight, it is really hard to do that and because I had no resistance from the person who was disabled, it was kind of a no-brainer for me.

Is this really the issue then, that the nurse educator described above offered no resistance to moving from teaching clinicals to being in the classroom? What if the nurse educator had wanted to continue teaching hospital clinicals to students or if the nursing school did not have anyone as well qualified as this educator to teach those clinicals? Why couldn't an aide or another nurse on the floor have shown the students how to lift or move a patient? Was the clinical instructor being valued more for the ability to show the mechanics of nursing than for what she could teach the students about being a nurse? This narrative recalls one described earlier about the termination of a nurse who was obese because she couldn't help a patient up off of the floor. As a profession, nursing continues to emphasize that it is our ability to think critically and intelligently and to make sound decisions that characterizes nurses. However, it appears that we contradict ourselves by saying that the nurse must also be able to lift and move patients.

A nurse who had recently graduated from nursing school suggested having disability insurance for nursing students because of the physical risk.

> Nursing students practice in environments where all of the risk is born by the students if they injure their back or have certain types of exposure ... unless it is reported immediately where there might be some sort of coverage, frequently it becomes a chronic disability. There is no compensation or any recognition of the impact of that on their future earnings, potential earnings.

An advanced practice nurse recalled injuring her back when she was working as an RN in the emergency department. She found that staff and administrator attitudes changed toward her as a result because people felt that she couldn't do her job. She tried to tell others that it was a safety issue for both nurses and patients to have to lift obese patients, especially those with tubes and other equipment. The physical risk from doing the job of a nurse exists for the bedside nurse, the nursing instructor, and even the student nurse. Should the inability to perform lifting and moving tasks preclude the opportunity to be a nurse or a nurse educator?

EVERYONE HAS THE POTENTIAL TO BE UNSAFE

Patient safety can be impacted by any number of things, too numerous to detail here. These have already been detailed by the Institute of Medicine (1999) in their report *To Err is Human*. There are obvious threats to safety such as medication errors and failure to follow aseptic technique when doing wound care or inserting intravenous lines, for example. However, there are more subtle ways in which a nurse could potentially jeopardize patient safety such as incompetence or a lack of knowledge regarding how to perform a procedure or care for a particular patient but failing to acknowledge that ignorance so that someone who is capable can do what needs to be done.

New graduates, nurses new to a particular field of nursing, and nurses new to a particular facility or organization might make mistakes because they are unfamiliar with the policies and procedures. This is not an acceptable excuse, however, because nurses are oriented by their organizations regarding policies and procedures and are expected to know and follow them. However, nurses often "float" to different areas in a hospital, particularly, and may not be as familiar with the procedures performed on that particular unit.

A nurse might jeopardize patient safety by taking shortcuts, by not following physician orders exactly or at the designated time. A nurse might forget to document something or not document it correctly, thereby leaving room for potential error.

It is interesting to note that when nurse managers talk of how nurses with disabilities might jeopardize patient safety, it is not those noted above that are discussed, which are conceivable for any nurse, but those which could seemingly be avoided by a little forethought and strategizing. In other words, the nurse with a disability might be assigned to do something else within that particular unit that would prevent the nurse from being in a position that would allow the disability to impact patient safety. The inability to do cardiopulmonary resuscitation (CPR) seems to be a common cause of concern.

CPR AND SAFETY

The issue of being able to pass the CPR exam has been raised in an earlier chapter. Inability to perform CPR is seen as a safety issue for patients and has been the cause of some nurses with disabilities not getting or keeping their jobs. It has been used as an excuse to terminate nurses.

> I took a recert [CPR] course. . . . The instructor flunked me because I couldn't get, supposedly of course, enough compressions and strong enough compressions on the manikin, no matter where the manikin was placed. So, he flunked me. And the employer said "Well, you can't work because you failed CPR." So, I went to the American Heart Association (AHA) a week later. They made a provision of putting the manikin at maybe six or eight inches lower for better compressions. Passed it with no sweat. Showed the employer the new certification and they said "No. We're terminating your services because you could not pass the CPR." . . . And even in their employee handbook [it] stated that anybody that failed a CPR test was to be suspended until [such] time they got a new certification done and they never took their own handbook into consideration.

This nurse was terminated and consequently couldn't pay her bills. At the time of the interview, her house was at risk of foreclosure. She sought legal counsel but could not afford to pay for it. This "depleted all my resources, insurance policies, everything, to keep current on my bills and my mortgage and I just can't do it anymore." Despite her difficulty with CPR and her slowed mobility, she was able to perform her work safely.

> I can get there in a timely manner and my bedside manner and my nursing skills are not compromised in any way at all. . . . My disability had no . . . interference with anything, interactions with the families, or patients, or other personnel I was working with.

Still, she was viewed as being potentially unsafe. "I can't hide [my disability]. It just takes me longer to get somewhere and they view that as something wrong and something that I can't do and it's a hazard to their requirements for patient care." . . . Although this nurse met the requirements for passing CPR by the AHA, her failure to pass CPR by the hospital's instructor, from her perspective, was used to terminate her. The fact that her disability did not otherwise impact her ability to provide quality care did not seem to matter.

Another nurse who couldn't do CPR because of knee problems decided on her own that she should leave nursing because the job is too physical.

> I can't do CPR because I can't get down on my knees.... So, I felt that I can't do nursing the way it should be done.... I don't want to put my patients at risk. I don't want to put anybody at risk.

She described having been a nurse for so long that, given an emergency situation, her knowledge of CPR would automatically kick in and she would do what she had to do. "I'm sure that would happen but I don't want to wait to see if that would happen." Yet being able to get to an emergency quickly, let alone the ability to perform CPR, seems to be a reason to not work in acute care situations for the nurse with a disability.

NURSES WITH DISABILITIES WORRY THAT THEY JEOPARDIZE SAFETY

Nurses with disabilities tend to be very concerned about jeopardizing patient safety. The nurse described above said that her doctor suggested she use a cane. Her response was: "How would that look as a nurse showing up with a cane where you're relied upon for emergencies. If you're relied upon for emergencies, you can't be using a cane." This nurse went further to say:

> I can't do nursing in the traditional sense because I think it's a liability for me and I don't want to jeopardize my patients.... I can't be depended upon. I'd be the first one to admit that ... so how could I in good conscience go and apply for a job and make people [think] "Oh, you know we have a nurse now and we're gonna count on her" and then all of a sudden for some reason they can't count on me. So that also is very humiliating, you know, to not be dependable.

This nurse was typical of the nurses with disabilities who worried that they would somehow hurt a patient because of their disability. They frequently removed themselves from nursing as a result. This seems a drastic and unnecessary response when the nurse could be redirected to another area of nursing, if necessary. Another nurse was very frank about this when asked if it is ever justifiable to prevent a nurse with a physical disability from working in a particular area of nursing:

> In the OR [operating room] if it was dangerous, if you couldn't move fast enough to get out of the way. Right now, I can't imagine that I would do OR.... I couldn't move fast enough to get out of the way and I would never endanger a patient's life.

He described discussing this issue with a friend who felt that as long as one was a fully trained nurse, one should be able to work. The nurse with the disability responded: "I said, that's narcissistic, that's putting yourself in front of the patient. I've worked in situations where you have to get your ass out of the way.... You run... and you cannot mess around. You're in a hurry." This nurse discussed a situation in which he had to give a patient an injection and was unable to give it the full amount of pressure required because of his lack of strength. As a result he decided "I'm going to stop, this is my last shot."

> I can't feel a thing... once I have gloves on, 'cause I rubbed the site, couldn't feel and I thought, "My hand, it's a little bit shaky, I can't feel." I had a hard time pinching the skin and I thought "That's it for me."... My arm has lost its ability to do that.... I don't believe I could start an IV now because of the [lack of] feeling. Why would [anyone] hire me? I don't think they should. I don't think I'd be safe. I know the stuff. I'm good, but I don't think that I would be safe and I just think you have to put the patient first.

This nurse may be accurate in thinking that he could not care for patients safely in certain settings but it seems unnecessary to lose his knowledge and expertise to the profession entirely. If he and others with disabilities felt comfortable seeking assistance to find a new position either within their current organization or somewhere else within nursing, the knowledge and expertise they have would not be wasted. One nurse described why it is so important to look beyond the disability to what the nurse can offer "What nursing brings to the table theoretically is decision making, clinical judgment, etc. It's what makes us different and you know that is something apart from how fast you move or how big you are."

A nurse with hand tremors that were unrelated to any disease process was sometimes viewed as a risk to patient safety but perhaps was more of a risk to her own safety. She had difficulty with needles and had stuck herself with unclean needles. In any case, she was told by Human Resources to see a neurologist to be sure she could perform all of her nursing duties safely. She did so and got a note from the neurologist saying that she could perform all of her duties safely.

> The only thing I really have trouble with doing that I honestly cannot do: I cannot carry those stupid Styrofoam cups, especially full of hot coffee, hot tea, anything like that I can't do it. . . . My boss was kinda like. . . . "You have to go down and see [Human Resources] because . . . there had been complaints about you not being able to perform your duties as a nurse so you need to [get] . . . a note from your neurologist saying that you can do everything." And I was like "Well, who was complaining?" You know, of course, they're not gonna tell you.

Interestingly, she asked that the facility get lids for the cups and in the 5 years since she had asked, they never got lids for the cups.

> I have burned myself. I've had blisters on my hands before from the coffee cups so I don't even usually try it anymore if I don't have a lid for it. . . . That's all I wanted. That's all I told Human Resources I wanted. Just get lids for the Styrofoam cups, please. That's the only thing I need so I can carry it to [the patient's] room. "Okay, we'll get it." No, haven't seen 'em.

On bad days, the nurse identified that she needed help with certain tasks but she knew her limitations and since the tremors were genetic and not disease related, she had no other neurological sequelae. Patients would ask her if she was nervous but never asked for a different nurse to perform their care. "Nothing's ever happened to any of my patients . . . but it's just . . . embarrassing I guess is the biggest thing." She did, however, often have to apologize to the doctors.

> I apologize to the doctors a lot . . . and they probably don't like that either but . . . if they're doing a culture or something and they have to put it in the tube and I'm holding the tube [and] if my hand moves a little bit then they miss it and then it's contaminated and they have to do it again.

A nurse who is in the capacity of supervisor or manager or nurse educator should be able to continue to make decisions or teach regardless of the physical disability. A nurse who walks slowly and has trouble walking long distances was told that despite her experience as a supervisor of a psychiatric unit, liability issues were potentially involved if she continued to work.

There are times I could get into a physical confrontation with a client, when they get into their confrontational mood—we are trying to be a restraint-free facility totally—[but] there are still going to be times when I may have to [handle] somebody . . .

However, she said that most of her job as supervisor involved decision making and felt that she could still be used in that capacity. She understood that she might be at risk if a psychiatric patient became confrontational and was willing to avoid being in that position as long as she could continue to stay in her supervisory role.

COMPENSATING

Many nurses are able to compensate for what they are no longer able to do in the traditional way. Sometimes, these compensations are met with collegial and administrative support but at other times, people are not comfortable having things done in a way that is different whether or not it is safe. A nurse with post polio syndrome described compensating safely for her limitations. Her colleagues and administrators were supportive of her efforts. Some nurses and physicians in a recent study comparing the work life experiences of physicians and nurses with disabilities (Neal-Boylan, 2012; Neal-Boylan et al., 2012) found that colleagues were discomfited by their methods of compensating and wanted them to do things the usual way.

THE SAFETY OF THE NURSE

Then there is the issue, not to be ignored, of the safety of the nurse. Often it is the nurse who, aware of his or her limitations verbalizes to administrators what may jeopardize their own safety and how the nurse might compensate for what they cannot do. Examples of nurses who might have their own safety compromised include the nurse who is immunosuppressed but is asked to care for an infectious patient or a nurse with musculoskeletal disabilities who might have a potential for falling. A nurse described earlier in this book who had severe allergies to perfumes is in jeopardy when staff, despite the facility's policy, wear heavy scents to work. A nurse with diabetes may need to eat their meals at regularly scheduled times to prevent illness. In instances such as these, the nurse becomes his or her own best advocate but sometimes they are penalized for raising the issue and consequently try to hide the disability (Chapter 3) as long as possible. In some cases, however, it is unsafe for them to hide the disability or chronic illness but they often risk discrimination or termination when they reveal it. Interactions with staff, administrators, and patients and the issue of nurse safety will be discussed further in Chapter 6.

THE PATIENT PERSPECTIVE

It is important that we not overlook the patient perspective regarding whether or not the nurse with a disability puts patient safety at risk. Interestingly, many people, when asked, don't seem to have any concerns about being taken care of by nurses with physical or sensory disabilities as long as they know how to do their jobs. Some do, however, express concern regarding receiving care from nurses with cognitive disabilities. This view espouses that as long as the nurse is competent, there is not a severe learning disability and the nurse is capable of following directions, then there is little concern, if any.

There is the opposing view, however, of some people who believe that being treated by a person with a disability poses a risk to the patient and may prevent the patient from getting the best treatment. This appears to be the case particularly in an emergency situation even if the person knows that the nurse is intellectually and emotionally competent. Interestingly, some people have said that while publicly they espouse the view that persons with disabilities should be treated just like everyone else is treated, they acknowledge that in a situation in which they are receiving care, they would prefer to receive care from a person without a physical or sensory disability over someone who had one. This perspective allows that even a person with a visual disability who cannot read the fine print in the chart or electronic medical record might need help from other nurses to ensure that they provide safe and appropriate care. This coincides with the "not in my back yard" mentality that is often used when people vote on new regulations in their own cities and states.

When asked how they felt about receiving care from a nurse with a physical or sensory disability, some patients commented that they are more concerned when the nurse cannot speak English because they might possibly not understand English or when the nurse is obese because it would be hard to accept their medical and health care advice. This also seems to be true for nurses who smoke or use drugs.

Year after year, nurses are noted to be among the most trusted professionals by the public. People expect nurses to role model healthful behaviors and they expect nurses to translate and interpret medical jargon and bad news for them. When a nurse cannot be understood or the patient worries that they cannot communicate with the nurse, this may be viewed as a handicap to receiving quality, safe care. If a nurse does not him- or herself ascribe to healthful behaviors, how is the patient to believe that they should do so or that it is possible to change their own behavior?

Perhaps nursing as a profession should focus more on rectifying the health behaviors of its own so that our current and future patients will continue to trust our judgment instead of on whether a nurse who has a disability should be held to a higher standard than nurses without visible disabilities.

It seems clear that nurses with disabilities are no more likely to jeopardize patient safety than nurses without disabilities. Nurses with disabilities seem, in general, to recognize on their own when they can no longer care for patients safely in a particular setting. They should be encouraged and directed to other possible uses for their expertise that will allow them to remain as paid members of the profession. The profession should be more vigilant about keeping nurses who cannot provide safe care because they lack sufficient knowledge or judgment rather than because of their physical or sensory disabilities.

REFERENCES

Institute of Medicine. (1999). *To err is human: Building a safer health system.* Washington, DC: National Academy Press.

Neal-Boylan, L., Fennie, K., & Baldauf-Wagner, S. (2011). Nurses with sensory disabilities: Their perceptions and characteristics. *Rehabilitation Nursing, 36*(1), 25–31.

Neal-Boylan, L., Hopkins, A., Skeete, R., Hartmann, S. B., Iezzoni, L. I., & Nunez-Smith, M. (2012). The career trajectories of health care professionals practicing with permanent disabilities. *Academic Medicine, 87*(2), 172–178.

Neal-Boylan, L. J. (2012). An exploration and comparison of the worklife experiences of registered nurses and physicians with permanent physical and/or sensory disabilities. *Rehabilitation Nursing, 37*(1), 3–10.

6

Nurses With Disabilities and the Health Care Environment

Sofia, a 56-year-old doctorally prepared advanced practice nurse (APN), was teaching lecture and clinical courses at a local university. She taught one of her classes in a large amphitheater. During class, she had to walk up and down the aisles to make eye contact with the students. This classroom was on the third floor of a building that was a quite a distance from her office. One day each week, Sofia took 10 undergraduate nursing students to a medical floor at the local hospital. In addition, she made site visits to the clinical placements of her nurse practitioner students. Sofia became paraplegic following a horseback riding accident and became confined to a wheelchair. While she was in the hospital, her colleagues covered her classes. When she returned from her rehabilitation she found that her office had been moved to the first floor of the academic building. This was helpful in allowing her to maneuver her wheelchair into her office but she was removed from the nursing offices and thus from her colleagues. She had previously enjoyed having them stop by and stopping by herself to chat when they weren't in class. She felt isolated. The Chair of her nursing department met with her shortly after her return to discuss her classes. The Chair told Sofia that she should be appropriately grateful as other faculty had worked hard to cover her classes and had to deal with increased stress as a result. She informed Sofia that she would no longer be taking the undergraduates to the hospital clinical but that she was needed to resume her other classes and to add a class teaching fundamentals of nursing to undergraduates to make up for not teaching the clinical course. When she asked the Chair why she could not continue to teach the clinical course as the hospital was completely accessible, she was told that since she could no longer lift or move patients, she should not be teaching a clinical course. Sofia argued that she could explain the mechanics of lifting and moving patients and have the students perform these tasks with the nurse's aides who worked on the hospital floor but the

Chair would not waver. Sofia resumed teaching her other courses despite the long distance in a wheelchair to the amphitheater. She also found that she could no longer climb the aisles of the amphitheater and asked to have her classroom moved. She asked to switch with another class that had approximately the same number of students. Sofia was advised to remain in the amphitheater where she would have to stay at the front while teaching the class. Sofia took over the Fundamentals of Nursing lab class for the colleague who had switched with her and took her clinical group to the hospital. Shortly after, her Chair asked to meet with her again. The Chair had heard from many of the students that Sofia was unable to demonstrate several of the fundamental skills to the students. Sofia again countered that she could explain the skills and that the students also had videos to watch to learn how to do the skills. Sofia explained that it was her feeling that she brought to her classes her experience and expertise in caring for patients beyond the physical skills and that students could still benefit from her knowledge even though she was limited physically. Sofia continued to make site visits to the clinical placements of her nurse practitioner students even though this involved frequently getting in and out of her car and maneuvering her way into various buildings. The next semester, the Chair did not allocate the Fundamentals class to Sofia and Sofia found that she was not given the usual choices given to faculty regarding which classes she wanted to teach.

Nurses with disabilities often encounter barriers to being able to perform their work and to integrate successfully and effectively within an organization. The environments in which they work, whether in a health care agency or a school of nursing, are not always amenable to navigation by a nurse with a disability. Further, the intangible aspects of the environment, such as the attitudes of colleagues and patients may not always conform to the expectations of the nurse with a disability.

Chapter 3 discussed how many nurses with disabilities tend to hide that they have a disability when this is possible to do because they fear that others will look at the disability and not at their nursing qualifications. Those who have had to reveal their disabilities have often felt that they received short shrift when they have gone for interviews before their interviewers have had the opportunity to learn about their qualifications for the job. In this chapter, nurses speak about the attitudes of others once they have the job, particularly after the disability compels the nurse to develop compensatory techniques or habits.

Nurses with disabilities often attempt to compensate for what they are unable to do in the usual way. Sometimes these attempts are applauded and at other times they are frowned upon. This is among the sometimes difficult interactions experienced by nurses with disabilities with colleagues and supervisors who may set unrealistic expectations of them above that of nurses without disabilities. However, there are also many positive interactions that these nurses experience and describe. Previous studies have found that collegial and administrative support are the most significant factors in having a nurse with disabilities stay in the job and/or in nursing.

This chapter discusses and describes some of those interactions, both positive and negative, including interactions with patients. The barriers that nurses with disabilities have identified as pivotal to whether or not they stay in their jobs or in nursing are revealed through the stories the nurses share. The attempts nurses make to compensate for what they cannot easily do because of their disabilities is demonstrated through the voices of nurses who have had both positive and negative work life experiences.

INTERACTING WITHIN THE HEALTH CARE ENVIRONMENT

Nurses with disabilities have both positive and negative interactions while working in the health care environment. Naturally, the perceptions of interactions may be colored by many factors beyond the question of disability. Nurses tend to work under a great deal of stress and it can be hard to distinguish whether someone is treating you in a certain way because of issues that revolve around your disability or whether they have a fundamental problem with your work ethic or the quality of your work. The narratives of the nurses in this chapter concern interactions that they perceived to be related to having a disability. However, it is important to recognize that there are two sides (sometimes more) to every story and that these are only the perceptions of the nurses with disabilities and not of their colleagues or managers.

Chapter 3 discussed why many nurses with disabilities hide their disabilities whenever possible. Once they are hired it is often necessary to wait until the nurse has gotten to know others in the facility and they know the quality of his or her work before they reveal the disability.

> I think the only person I've mentioned it to is the medical assistant that I work with most closely who works with me every day and we talked a lot about our lives in general and we have a very supportive relationship of one another, so I felt like I could say that and she wouldn't view it as I'm looking to get out of something but rather she'd take it as understanding if something came up.... [for example if] I told her I was having a bad day, she

would take it for what it was, not try to second guess what that was about. . . . This job is still so new to me that I haven't had a lot of conversation [about it]. . . . So, I think I would probably have that conversation but it really depends on who I was trying to talk to about it, whether [it would] be some[one] that I felt would be understanding, would find me valuable enough that they wanted to be accommodating. . . . If you've been there long enough they can look at my body of work and say she's a productive member of the team, it's worth trying to accommodate her in order to keep her on.

One nurse who had a variety of health issues that contributed to disability did not feel that she received accommodations despite having worked at the facility for a long time and having made a significant contribution. The nurse who was allergic to perfumes and scents tried to talk to administrators about the problem especially since their institution's policy was that staff did not wear perfumes or anything scented.

[The administrator] . . . wore a little bit of perfume and some of her staff did and it was really low scent but they're not around the other people. But when I go up to complain or say something, I'm around them and then they had a new [nurse] come in and she wore unscented everything. But they said, it's a hard thing to enforce that no scents be used because they've got scented soaps, they've got scented shampoos . . . You don't have to smell like a rose coming to work you know what I mean?

In this case, the nurse had a negative interaction because she did not feel that administrators took her seriously with regard to how significant scents and perfumes could be to causing allergic reactions in her or in patients and visitors. Interestingly, the institutional policy spoke against using scented products but this was typical of a rule that was not rigorously followed because it was simply too difficult to enforce. This same nurse also had a disability that affected one of her arms and she discussed her interactions regarding trying to get accommodations so she could work.

I asked for a chair with arms on it for years. . . . I said . . . keep your arm hanging bent all day. It's heavy. . . . I don't have to hold it there, it's bent. I don't have a choice, but it hurts. And I asked, and I asked. [The supervisor] said "You should have put it in writing. I said "well, I emailed [and] she said "No, put it in a formal letter." Well the atmosphere is . . . very pleasant . . . where I love everyone . . . I get along. I've been there almost since it opened, you just don't complain. It's almost like: don't ask, don't talk.

The nurse clearly needed a chair with arms, on the surface a simple request. However, she was told that a formal letter was required and still she did not get the chair. She was hesitant to push the issue because she liked her work environment and felt that everything would run smoothly if no one made waves. This nurse also asked about getting a wooden desk instead of the large secretary desk she had so she could work more comfortably.

> Now I have almost no feeling in my left hand and I don't type well anyway and in doing that, I have this corner desk so I'm sitting at an angle with the computer at an angle because I have to type.... I said if I had a wooden desk instead of this big secretary desk, which I don't need anyway, I could at least put the whole desk at an angle, push back the computer and be straight because I'm all askew, plus I have to elevate my foot. I brought in a stool from home. [Administration said] "Oh well, we'll look into that." It's been almost a year, "we've been looking into it." Email after email, they just keep giving me this "Well, we're working on it." I finally said to my supervisor ... this is against the law. ... It's a huge issue anyway. But the point, I think, is that I feel really badly about it and don't get why and I feel like I represent so many of my patients and veterans who come back without a limb and they're made to feel terrible ... I feel like I'm asking for the moon. I'm the only person with a metal desk by the way. ... But why do I have to beg?

This narrative raises several concerns. Firstly, people with disabilities are supposed to be given any reasonable accommodation and a chair with arms and a wooden desk that she could use to arrange her work area in an ergonomic way, seem reasonable accommodations to make. Despite her longevity at the facility (which should not have to be a factor), she still could not get anyone to respond to her requests. Finally, this nurse raises the issue of how others, such as veterans, with disabilities are treated. Her narrative exposes the fact that as a nation we have not been keen to recognize people with disabilities as people first and that they have the same rights as everyone else to expect to be provided with the tools they need to perform their work. This nurse had also tried to negotiate for a parking space close to the door of the facility as she has trouble walking.

> There's one handicap parking space and it's near the ... entrance. It was made for a physician who died.... It's usually taken by a patient.... So I usually get there [early] enough so I can get a decent place but I cannot leave for lunch or lose my place. And I have to park, especially in the winter, close enough to the door because ... the halls are really long and I can't walk really long

hall[s]. The only other handicap place is near the front door and I've asked a couple of times and they say in order to get handicap parking, you have to go to city council and it's a very big deal. So, this winter I'm terrified because I'm scared in the winter anyway [in case] I fall. . . . So, this winter, I'm going to have to get to work really early and I will never be able to leave at lunch or I will lose my place. I can't walk on slippery places . . . that just seems wrong.

This narrative exemplifies a not uncommon situation in which the person with a disability must make sacrifices in order to obtain the accommodations he or she need to do their work. In this case this nurse must arrive early to get a parking space close to the building and she cannot move her car during the day. Other people can come and go and leave for lunch, but this nurse risks losing her parking space if she does so. This is clearly unfair. The nurse consulted a lawyer who advised her to write a formal letter saying that the facility is required to provide her with a handicap parking space that will be available to her and an ergonomically correct desk. When asked how she thought the letter would be received she replied:

Horribly and I will be perceived as a pain in the ass. . . . I gotta look for another place to work. . . . In my case . . . I have to work harder or have to apologize for a handicap. I am pulling my weight, more than pulling my weight, and doing my job, not a bit affected by the handicap. My job is not affected. Getting to my desk, sitting at my desk, the mechanics, period, are affected, that's it. How simple. It may cost a few pennies but I am more than making up for it with my work and its quality.

This nurse discussed having her annual review with her supervisor and having her disability mentioned as part of the review. "I just think . . . getting a review . . . I got full raise and lots of praise and it was a great review, but I think that to mention a handicap specifically should not be okay." Often, people with disabilities are seen as troublemakers if they make too many requests for accommodations or they complain about not being provided with the reasonable accommodation to which they are entitled. Advocating for oneself may be seen as complaining, which in turn appears to lead to efforts to push the person out of the job without allowing it to appear that this has anything to do with their disability.

A nurse who suffered from severe and limiting back pain had a different experience and spoke of receiving support from the nurses and certified nurse's aides (CNA) on her floor.

They were really great, actually. Other nurses would help me out. . . . I just couldn't roll a patient by myself. I couldn't help a patient get out of bed.... Though that wasn't one of my strict job [requirements], I was responsible for the patent, but the CNAs I worked with were fantastic. They didn't make me feel bad. They didn't get cranky or give me any crap about it.... I always made a point to say "I'm really sorry that I can't do that for you. "... They were really nice to me, so it was good.... My supervisors were nice and no one gave me a hard time at all.

Another nurse who worked on an orthopedic floor felt that her colleagues were also very supportive.

The aides would come and if they knew I could not do a heavy lift they'd come and help me or say "I know you have to get Mrs. X up, why don't you let me know when you're ready and I'll give you a hand, get an extra body in here to help."... The staff was very cohesive, it was a good group to work with.

It was interesting in the studies that were done of nurses with disabilities to find that nurses who became disabled but who worked on orthopedic units were provided with more support than were nurses who worked on other floors or units and became disabled. This is likely because orthopedic nurses work day-to-day with people who have suffered injury or alterations in mobility or function and are practiced at helping people to emphasize what they *can* do as opposed to what they cannot do. It is also interesting that, frequently, when nurses with disabilities spoke of from whom they got support, it was more often from the nurse's aides than from their nurse colleagues or administrators. This nurse felt that her colleagues were supportive of her because it was an orthopedic floor and because her head nurse set the tone for how they would treat her.

The head nurse stepped in and said ... we're going to take care of our own. So [I] definitely had the cohesion of the staff and support of the head nurse. I think that was most important. I think if she had set the tone differently, staff would have responded differently.

It has become clear, through the research that has been done thus far, that having supportive colleagues and administrators makes all the difference in whether a nurse stays on the job. This is a perfect example of how the head nurse set the tone for the staff that the unit would support the nurse who had become disabled.

This same nurse, however, went on to say:

I sensed frustration on the administration side that they were having difficulty trying to figure out what to do with me....

> I couldn't always work charge [nurse] because there were other people that were qualified to work charge as well and for me to take over the charge position, there were senior people who wanted to do that as well. So, when I was not working charge and having to work staff nursing and then [having] them see me incapacitated at the end of the day . . . there were some gentle suggestions that staff nursing might not be a good idea. . . .

She said that despite working in that hospital for 10 years, no one stepped forward to try to help her find another nursing position within the hospital. She lamented that there is no standard mechanism in place to help the nurse with a disability return to work.

> Nursing is a very hard job and people have to be in top notch shape to be able to do it. I think once somebody's injured . . . the mechanism is not in place for people to return to that work and still function as a viable member of the team. . . . [It is seen as taking] away from the ability of the team to do a complete job. . . . I've worked in enough places now that I think flexibility can be worked into even a nursing unit where you're giving care to patients on the floor.

This is a common theme that echoes throughout the stories told by nurses with disabilities. Most typically, nurses are not given any guidance or assistance to find other jobs within the health care agency or within nursing. This nurse went into home health nursing and found little difficulty or resistance related to having a disability.

> I was able to drive to the client's home and sit down in their living room or at their kitchen table . . . and do what needed to be done. Any standing I did would be to get up to get something out of my bag or to kneel down to do a dressing change or to assess . . . but it was limited time spent on my feet. [It was] a lot of time driving around in my car and sitting down and talking to people, a lot of teaching in home health. [Administration and staff] knew ahead of time that I had this disability and it was not a problem if I needed to bring my cane . . .

In this case, home health nursing turned out to be a good career move for this nurse.

A hospital nurse described an interaction she had with her manager:

> One morning I came in to work and it was one of the bad days with my hand and I was actually scheduled to have an MRI or

something and the [manager] told me [she] wanted to meet with me.... So that day, I was spoken to in a conference room and I was very fragile at that point ... I was worried about what was going on with my body and this one manager ... had this sheet of just ... crazy, ridiculous issues and I remember getting teary at one point.... One of the things was that "You're always concerned about whose gonna be the late nurse when you come in." We all had schedules, so we knew ahead of time who was gonna be the late nurse but being a late nurse on that unit could mean that you would work a 12- to 13-hour shift if it ran over. I got teary at that point and I said "You know I have issues with my health and there's no one else that has to be vigilant about those issues than me." ... They were awful. They were cold. They were nonresponsive. They were mean. It was awful. It was awful.

Not being able to work all different shifts is a common problem among nurses with disabilities. Often fatigue overwhelms them and they cannot work more than their usual shift or work at night. Others often see this as shirking their responsibilities or as not being a good team player. A nurse who worked nights, however, talked of the support she received from her coworkers and speculated that that this might have to do with working the night shift. "The girls on the night shift with me are very good about it and they're helpful.... If I say "I really can't do this today," they'll [say] "Alright well, I'll do that and you do this for me." She talked about being perfectly capable of doing her job but of having to try to get used to staff, physicians, and patients staring at her and automatically assuming that she could not do her job just because of her tremors.

They might ask somebody else to help them do something instead of me. One of the girls might just say "Oh, I'll do it." They're probably helping me but sometimes I [say] "I can do that. You know you don't need to go and do that for me." They might not even do it for that reason, but just the fact that they'll [say they'll do it]. . . . They go and take care of it. I'll [think] "Why did they offer to do that? Why couldn't I do it? They don't think I'm good enough to do it? Why couldn't I do it?" ... But a lot of that could just be me ... I should probably just let it go.... I try to make light of it the best I can because there's nothing else you can do about it.... If you can't laugh at yourself, who can you laugh at? I've never hurt any of my patients . . .

Another nurse with diabetes told her colleagues and supervisors that she could not do any lifting "They sort of scowled but that's where I have to take the initiative and I have to find out how to get the mission done." When asked if she had been giving any accommodations she responded:

> I think in the [patient] assignment sometimes they try and there are always difficult patients that are potentially combative and I think they try to give me a sensible patient load and not take advantage in any way or overload me.

But this nurse believes that it is the nurse's responsibility to ask for what she or he needs and to make it happen.

> It's up to you. You have to take the responsibility to say I need my lunch break, I need to go. We have tried to work out a buddy system so I can report to another RN and she covers my patients so I can take a break. If there is a dispute that everyone wants to go at a similar time . . . if you work collegially with your colleagues, you can work it out. . . . A disabled person has to look to their own adaptations. You can't expect the work place to facilitate every need. You have got to be creative.

Another nurse with minimal function in one knee talked about the need to lift patients despite that requirement not being listed in her job description. Sometimes she can count on help from nurse's aides and other times she cannot.

> There's an interesting relationship between techs (medical technicians) and nurses as I'm sure there are everywhere, but I would say there's decent amount of support if you need it. Unfortunately, It's not always available so . . . I was getting put in some interesting situations where I was left responsible for complete total patient care of somebody that was much heavier than I was able to support. I just wasn't able to do it. I ended up having to leave the patient and get some help.

Another nurse said that having an environment over which you have some degree of control can help the nurse with disabilities work effectively: "That's my difficulty. I am okay in my environment that I can control, but when you heap stress on me to produce, I can't do it and yet that's what I try doing." This nurse had had a stroke and had difficulty communicating easily.

> People don't even wait for you to respond conversationally. They give you a second and if [you] don't come back with something, they either answer for you or they're moving on.

This nurse who had been a master's prepared administrator with many years of nursing and executive experience talked of her determination to go back to work after suffering a stroke and had been told that she could not.

> It's not an open, loving environment with somebody standing there saying "come on back" to the nurse that's disabled. [Instead] it's "Can't you find something else to do or go to work for somebody else? We really don't want you back." There's a difference in the attitude. No one would have ever said to me "Are you up to the task?" before the stroke.

She spoke of the attitude of her nurse colleagues after her stroke:

> They were very angry with me, extremely angry that I had the audacity to have this happen. I've actually had people say to me "You need to get yourself together. Just pull yourself together. It's been long enough."

It continues to confound nurses who shared their stories that while nurses will do almost anything to care for their patients, they will not show the same concern or compassion for their colleagues. One nurse was given light duty and a sedentary job while recovering from surgery. She was doing paperwork that needed to be done but despite that, it was not looked upon favorably by her colleagues.

> They've flat out told me that they believe it's favoritism that I get this cushy desk job because now I have an office with a desk and my own computer and they believe that I'm just let[ting] go of these responsibilities, which I understand. They've been left short staffed.... [That's] 40 hours of nursing time that's not been filled so they're working short pretty much always.

The work that this nurse was doing was vital to the functioning of the unit and if she hadn't been doing it, either someone else would have needed to do it or it wouldn't have gotten done. It seemed a perfect fit to give her the desk work while she was on light duty. Yet other staff resented her for it and she was not acknowledged as the person doing this work or given credit for what she accomplished. Even though the work continued beyond her physical need for light duty, she was not given a formal position or title.

> I think there's two issues: They see that I have something that I contribute despite my disability, so in that sense I think that

> they're able to say yes, we recognize that you have this problem and we're gonna try to help you out but it's not gonna be at the cost of the having to draw any attention to it. So I feel like they're shoving me under the table, like we're just not gonna talk about the fact that X's got this problem and that's why she can't do nursing work. Instead, we're gonna flood her with these responsibilities that get her seen and heard so that this looks like she's contributing, but we're not gonna actually bring it to the higher up levels.

One nurse described receiving verbal abuse from a member of the staff when she tried to get access to patient charts. He would barricade himself at a desk with the charts and she could not get around him because she used a walker. He refused to move and give her access and told her how much he disliked her when she finally left the job. When this nurse talked to attorneys about her experience working as a nurse with a disability they said "You'll never be able to prove subjective reasons why you're not hired but we get plenty of other nurses that come in with disabilities and they say the same exact thing." Conversely, another nurse who had joint pain and had trouble reaching things that were high up said that she felt supported.

> I may ask them for the fourth time to get something down from high up but they don't come at me like ". . . why don't you just get a stool?" They don't hold anything against me when I have to ask for help.

Clearly, attitudes and interactions are going to be influenced by many things other than whether or not a nurse has a disability. The awareness one has about disability, the general work load, the tone set by the manager are only some of the factors that can influence how a nurse with a disability perceives themselves to be treated in the health care environment. However, it is also clear that if reasonable accommodation can be made it must be made and that it is only right and fair to have a conversation with the nurse with the disability to explore the areas in which they feel they might need some help. In return, they might be able to take over some tasks that others do. It is important that a supportive tone be set by administrators so that staff will be more inclined to be supportive.

A nurse with rheumatoid arthritis said that her colleagues knew about the disease and were largely supportive.

> I've always been pretty open about it. I think in that position there were a few people who definitely didn't understand why I was having difficulty doing certain types of things. I think that my manager was pretty understanding. He was very willing to work with me and the majority of people I worked with there were.

> [There were] just one or two people who I felt like really didn't understand and expected me to do more than I was able in some situations. . . . I did have issues . . . some of the higher up management really didn't understand and I really had to fight as far as ADA type compliance, compliance with medical leave, that kind of thing and so I had to educate myself and then educate them on what those types of requirements were.

INTERACTIONS WITHIN THE ACADEMIC ENVIRONMENT

Many nurses with disabilities go back to school and obtain higher degrees. Others work in the academic environment as nurse educators. It is interesting to compare and contrast the experiences of the students with those of the faculty. There are other published sources that focus specifically on the experience of the nursing student with a disability. That is not the focus of this book. However, it is worthwhile to explore how the experiences of the students and the faculty sometimes differ. One nurse who discovered she had a severe latex allergy while still a student said that when she was taken to the emergency department where she was diagnosed with the allergy, a nurse came in to see her and told her she was nuts to consider pursuing a career as a nurse.

> I am disheartened by the lack of understanding of disabilities and the lack of support I have encountered from nurses in the practice setting (Neal-Boylan, 2012; Neal-Boylan et al., 2012) The nurse in the ER and the nurse performing the employee physical at that hospital [where] I was first hired at. I think that their, how should we say, lack of education, lack of knowledge to give it a nursing diagnosis . . . contributes greatly to the inability to effectively integrate nurses with disabilities into the clinical practice setting. At the same time, I am heartened by the incredible support of academic faculty who were able to recognize that nursing goes beyond hands-on care and were able to and tended to nurture me and foster my growth as a nursing professional despite that very great disability. I guess the experience has been very skewed and almost dramatically opposed depending on what type of nursing professional I was articulating with at that particular time.

Another nurse told how she needed to use crutches while a graduate student in nursing school and felt generally accepted there.

> I was accepted into a nursing program and there was one person who, she was a member of the faculty, did not believe that I could do it, did not believe that I belonged there, did not believe that

I deserved a spot there. She was ultimately dismissed. [Otherwise] I was very well accepted. You kind of get that look like "How can you do this?" but once they get to know me they see that it is not a problem.

Another nurse, while a graduate nursing student had a different experience while in school.

One of the problems that I was having was completing assignments. It was *very* . . . difficult for me to sit at a computer and concentrate and type, just sitting there typing was difficult. I didn't have a laptop and even sitting in a comfortable place with a laptop was also painful and difficult so I asked for assistance on the time frame of handing in assignments and one professor—I spoke with her about what the problem was and what I was doing to fix it and about the kind of help I was getting and about getting an extension—and she forgot that we talked about it. And another professor just said no. I asked if I could do some extra assignments. . . . One professor did give me an extension on a paper. . . . When I spoke with my advisor about all of that . . . that I tried to keep the professors up to date and tried to keep her informed and that I tried to tell them early and tried to tell them what was going on. . . . she said that I couldn't come back to school and that I couldn't get any help at all unless I registered with the office for students with disabilities. My first response was, why didn't you suggest that when I asked for help and my second response was: Wow, am I disabled? I didn't think of myself as disabled. I thought of myself as having a back injury. . . . I didn't know that the office for students with disabilities would support people with a back injury. I thought it was for people that are blind or deaf or in a wheelchair, like permanently for life disabled. So, I was confused about why nobody said that before I failed the class. . . . I thought, well I specifically asked you for help, why couldn't you have told me then? They responded no, we can't make accommodations for you unless you apply to this department. When I did get disability (through the office on student disability), I did get accommodations.

It is true that students are expected to apply through the university's department or office of student disability to get accommodations for classes. However, it is interesting to note that this graduate student was not aware that the office existed, that she needed to apply to it to get an accommodation or that she would even be considered to have a disability. As faculty, it is easy to assume that students will be aware of the existence of the office, as most universities require a blurb about the office of student disability to be inserted into their syllabi so that students are aware. However, if a student doesn't think of herself as disabled or if faculty don't bother to have a conversation with the student to explain what qualifies a student for possible accommodation, then it may be unreasonable to expect even a graduate student, let alone an undergraduate student, to understand that they must apply for accommodations. In this case, the nurse claims that she told faculty about her physical problems on numerous occasions in person and through email and that no one told her she needed to apply officially for accommodations until she failed the class.

The nurse sought help from the office on student disability and did receive accommodation but was now fearful of informing her professors about it.

> You apply to that office, you have an interview with them, you have to explain what's going on. . . . I told the director of that department what had happened . . . and how I had been treated and that I was kind of afraid it would happen now, that I didn't want to walk through that door, that it made me a little panicky. . . . She said now that you have been approved and we are going to see what type of accommodations we can give you, you are going to have to talk to them and tell your professors what is going on and this is your accommodation, whatever it is. I was kind of scared of that and I didn't want to talk to them at all because I didn't think they were very nice to me. So she agreed to write a letter and send it to . . . all of my professors. . . . My primary accommodation was just to get comfortable. I got an office chair and it was in the classroom just for me and I would sit in it and [one professor] asked me if I would need special testing accommodations . . . and I said no, I should be fine with this seat and . . . I can do it for the rest of this class . . . thanks so much for asking.

Once again, providing the right kind of chair seems like a simple accommodation to make so that a student can sit comfortably in class. Yet, due to poor communication and an apparent lack of willingness on the part of faculty to simply try to find out if anything as simple as a different type of chair would help this student, the student had to fail a class and seek the help of the office on student disability to get a chair she could sit in comfortably. She contrasted her experiences working as an RN versus her experience in graduate school.

> It's been a 50/50 shot whether you're accepted by peers or not. . . . I was lucky to have the nurses in my job be very supportive. If I had worked there long term and kept being unable to do things,

> I don't know if it would have been more grueling for them, if they had to pick up the slack ... but it was only a matter of [a few] months that I was actually still working there but as far as the nursing profession in academia, I think they're the most uncompassionate people I have ever met. . . . I had an awful, just awful experience at the university with this issue . . . Just professor after professor after professor being uncaring . . . we could care less if anything is harder for you. They say they want to help but they don't want to help . . . I had a handful that were really nice and supportive and I could tell that they really wanted me to graduate . . . but the rest of them, it was really pathetic.

This episode made the graduate student aware that she was considered disabled, at least as far as the university was concerned and it was a revelation to think of herself as disabled.

> I kind of claimed that title, if you will. You know, before that happened, before I had to apply to the disability office, I just thought of myself as having a fixable temporary back injury, like people have back injuries all of the time. . . . It really made me feel like I was falling into that slot of being disabled. I felt kind of helpless . . . like I had just been labeled that I was different that I needed help. . . . When I . . . told them that I couldn't get any help from my professors and from my advisor, I felt like they didn't care one way or another if I got help, if I dropped out. They didn't care if I finished the program, basically. I felt a little like I was forgiven because I was disabled now. [Prior to that time], I really thought they thought I was just an idiot in many ways because I wasn't telling the truth because I wasn't good enough to finish.

When this nurse completed her studies and was certified as a nurse practitioner she had this to say about how her disability affected her work: "I think it makes me a better practitioner that I have had these problems. . . ." The idea of gaining empathy as a result of having a disability seems fairly common. Many nurses said that this was an unexpected positive aspect of having a disability and working as a nurse.

A nurse with a disability who worked as nursing faculty commended other nurses who work in the academic environment for their supportive and helpful interactions. This nurse educator typically took nursing students to a third world country every year to work with the people there.

> I've been impressed that the university, that they were willing, that they didn't try to ask me not to go. I've been surprised that they've

been . . . pretty sympathetic and also, the dean was genuinely very helpful in terms of helping me implement my clinicals and stuff like that. . . . They have been very good at helping me with classroom issues. . . . Teaching in some classrooms is easier than teaching in other classrooms, it's hard for me to switch buildings, things like that. For example . . . I have to teach . . . on the fifth floor of another building so I have to get all of the equipment over there, get mobilized and that sort of thing. They have always been very good at trying to make adjustments and they encourage me.

This nurse educator went on to describe the challenges that can occur within the academic environment for a nurse with a disability.

The person most logical to share [information about] my disability with was the chairperson. That hasn't been so comfortable because anything I couldn't do had an impact on her and she wanted decisions made in advance at times when it wasn't always convenient to make those decisions, but I will say that they were pretty good about doing that.

Another nurse educator who has chronic pain from a car accident described retuning to the classroom.

So when I came back to work . . . I found it was more difficult to [teach in a classroom] . . . because I wasn't able to really move my neck in such a way that . . . if a student asked a question . . . and they were way back in the class—it was an auditorium style classroom—then I literally . . . had to change my position so I could look directly at the student. . . . It affects me in the classroom because I'm used to standing when I lecture and being very interactive, walking up and down steps in the auditorium if I have that classroom and I'm really not able to do that because I have some injuries around balance. . . . The potential of falling . . . has interfered with my teaching style. . . . I think even in terms of being able to write on the board or use the PowerPoint, there is a difference in my ability to do that comfortably. . . . In terms of my clinical work, it hasn't really impacted that except for fatigue level. . . . I have to walk a lot. . . . When I have pre- and postconference, the students sit either in a circle or at a long table. If it's in a circle, it's not as manageable because it's hard for me to turn my neck in such a way that I can really do the kind of one-to-one that I need to do.

Regarding working with students in the classroom, this nurse educator likes to use role play to illustrate important points and has tried bringing students to the front of the classroom instead of walking to where the students are sitting as she had previously done.

> Students are generally uncomfortable with that. They would prefer not being in front of the class and what they consider to be making a fool of themselves, which of course they're not . . . So I've had [to] accommodate that way. . . .

Another nurse educator spoke of being in the hospital after her disabling injury and not being visited by her faculty colleagues.

> I would've done the same thing if it was one of my colleagues and the schedules are busy and hectic and people probably plan to do it or wanted to do it. I don't think that they really have any idea of the way in which it affected me personally. . . .

She described how she was treated differently since her disabling condition. "They don't treat me like I'm anyone different but . . . I just feel like the step-child."

This nurse educator was told she should "be considerate of the faculty who took over for you and managed your advisees" while she was in the hospital. The nurse educator found this offensive particularly as she had thanked faculty for their support. She felt that she was being made to feel guilty by being in the hospital. She had received messages while still in the hospital asking when she would be back.

INTERACTIONS WITH PATIENTS

Nurses with disabilities get mixed responses from patients when patients realize that the nurse has a disability. Sometimes patients feel that the nurse knows how they feel as patients with chronic illnesses or disabilities. At other times, patients want their nurses to be without blemish so the patient can feel confident that nothing regarding their own care is missed.

Some nurses explain their disability to their patients so the patients understand that it won't affect the care the nurse provides. Typically nurses are not supposed to discuss their own problems with patients. One nurse gave an example: "Patients would say, 'Does your arm bend?' or 'How'd you do that?' and you really aren't supposed to share much of [your]self and I was able to."

This nurse who had been in an accident and had had many stitches in her face was able to empathize with a patient and explain to a patient and her child that things would get better.

> [I was at a] ... playground. [There was] a woman [who] had a little girl there who was ravaged on one side of her face and I said, "May I tell you something? ... I just want you to know I had over 100 stitches here and many here" and she just burst into tears. "So, trust me, your daughter is going to recover because ... she's going to heal. Keep her out of the sun, use vitamin B, trust me." And she was just so thankful. That's happened on [hospital] units. I've said to parents, "Can you see scars on my face? ... You think I just look horrible? No. Trust me, your kid is going to heal much better than this." ... However, I had a couple of charge nurses take issue with me sharing anything personal. "This is not about you." I know that, but trust me, I would have done anything to have somebody tell me that you can recover. ...

Patients may recognize that the nurse can be more empathetic with the patient if they have their own health problems but it is important that the nurse is careful to not call attention to him-/herself and take the focus from the patient. One nurse practitioner commented that having a disability

> can really strengthen the patient nurse relationship. If they know that you really understand, they will be more likely to talk to you and take your advice. ... It makes me a better nurse practitioner. I think I'm very compassionate about problems and just counseling patients.

Another nurse practitioner who came into nursing with a physical disability requiring that she be in a wheelchair commented:

> Patients actually have been incredible. ... That is one thing that surprised me when I became a nurse was how wonderful the patients are. Going in, I was expecting that people would be afraid or they'd be concerned that I wouldn't be safe or that I couldn't take care of them but it's been the total opposite. They've been absolutely amazing. ... I don't even have to ask them sometimes. ... "Can you move your head a little lower so I can use the stethoscope?"; they do it automatically. So the patients have been really good, almost too good sometimes where I have to say "It's okay I can do this and you don't need to get up and you don't need to hand me that." Sometimes, they almost want to overcompensate.

A nurse with a hearing disability said that he has had to instruct patients about his disability so they don't think he is ignoring them.

> I [have to tell them] if you tap me on the shoulder or something, then fine, I'll know ... I'm not ignoring you. ... That has caused a few problems and of course [there is added] stress ... for the patient and the family. They can get really annoyed.

Having experienced a chronic illness or disability can give the nurse an advantage over other nurses because she or he has some understanding of what the patient is experiencing and can anticipate the patient's needs and fears. One nurse said regarding having a disability and the patient relationship:

> I think [having a disability] gives me a really key advantage in that I have been in that bed so many times as a patient ... literally over and over and over, that I can see, I guess, the psychosocial side of it more and I think I am a very empathetic nurse. I think that I am a very caring nurse and [the other nurses] always tease me that I spend more time in the room than I do in the nurse's station and that's my whole point, I want the person in the bed to feel that they are not isolated because I have had experiences when I was in the hospital and I was terrified and I just felt like they just checked on me once a shift and that was it and I didn't want to ever do that to someone else.

This nurse uses a crutch to walk and says that she teases patients about the strength she has gained in her arms as a result. "I have some [patients] that have [said] 'Oh, you poor thing, I don't want to bother you' and then I tease them, of course and it's like 'Here, feel these arm muscles. I've got the strongest arm muscle you'll ever see.'"

Some patients may not mention the nurse's disability simply because they choose to focus on the nurse's expertise in providing their care. Patients don't typically want to hear about other people's health problems when they are dealing with their own and that seems reasonable. One nurse with arthritis and joint pain said:

> I've never had a single patient say anything to me. ... I think they're just grateful just to have nursing care. ... I treat them with respect, they treat me with respect. I mean, I think it's the way I approach them too. I don't try to carry myself and walk the way I walk just to bring attention to myself. ... I'm not moaning all about my pain ... even though I am [in pain], so ... people don't see me in that role, I don't think, as being handicapped.

Another nurse with benign hand tremors spoke of being teased by other nurses and patients and that she would typically take this as good-natured ribbing but there were times when she would not feel like being teased and get upset.

> On the days that [my disability] is bad, if I hear more than one comment in a shift, then I get mad. I can handle one, that's okay. You can say something once, that's fine but then after that.... [If] it's the girls (other staff) that are teasing me about it, I don't care, but [when] five patients tell me more than once, then it bothers me.... I guess I should be more open with my patients before I even start anything but I don't want to tell them about it if I don't need to.

A nurse with a lower extremity amputation commented:

> [People] are understandably curious. It's almost ubiquitous, people will say how did this happen? Some people are uncomfortable because I think they sort of reflect upon their own body image and seeing somebody else's body image different or altered in an uncomfortable way makes them sort of uncomfortable. I think it had a great deal more to do with their discomfort and embarrassment than mine. Actually it's neat working with the kids. Kids are very curious and ... it's very rewarding actually to say "You know, this leg got so sick it couldn't be saved but look at this device that helps me do the same things you can do!" It's like oh wow, this is neat. But it's the parents who seem to be uncomfortable more often.

In certain settings, it might behoove the nurse to admit to the disability so that others around her or him can offer to help when necessary. A nurse educator spoke of student responses to her disability:

> I just mention it in class that this is the situation why I might not be standing a regular way or that I might need to turn rather than to turn my neck, [I] turn my body.... Some of the students in clinical and in other situations have said to me if you need help let me know or they've offered to help and I've thanked them and other than pushing the door open for me, I'm not sure what they could do.... They have much more protection [in their] handbook around disabilities than [faculty] do....

COMPENSATIONS/ACCOMMODATIONS

Many nurses with disabilities learn to compensate for what they cannot do in the usual way. This often works well but colleagues and patients may be skeptical and uncomfortable. Some nurses are asked right away about the accommodations they will need. Others have to request accommodations and in doing so, educate others about what it's like to work with a disability. Not everyone is supportive of providing accommodations even if they are reasonable.

A nurse who only had full use of one arm said:

> I learned to compensate. I got the impression [that] staff weren't really happy about that. . . . They didn't think I could manage it and they didn't like it, I know. I just remember them behaving negatively, not patients, not doctors because I was pretty good at identifying people who needed care.

Some colleagues and administrators are supportive of nurses using accommodations and others are less so.

> I didn't even have the keyboard when I first started here because I said from the beginning . . . I really have a problem . . . in a flat keyboard situation and at the time my director said no problem and they ordered it for me. I mean, heck, forty or sixty dollars or whatever it was wasn't a big deal. I was willing to pay for it if I had to but I did not have to do that.

An advanced practice nurse who used a wheelchair said that she was asked about the accommodations she would need early on:

> So after I was hired, I met with the nursing supervisor and she sat down with me and she said, let's try our best to anticipate anything you might need and we went through the whole clinical [setting] and each room and we talked about how I'd be able to maneuver in each room, whether one room or another room would be better for me to see patients in, heights of where the gloves are kept, where the sharps [box is], things like that that I would need access to in the room and how I'd be able to sort of negotiate the exam table. . . . I have absolutely no problem discussing any kind of accommodation need with any of my supervisors.

This APN talked of the compensations she had had to make to do her job.

> Someone shows me how to do something and then I have to figure out how I'm going to do it because [the way] I'm gonna do it isn't necessarily the same way that they do it. I just need to reach the same ends without hurting the patient, obviously. Someone will

show me something and I have to work it through in my head how this would work for me, how I'm gonna get the same result knowing my capacity for physical strength, mobility, etc. What's gonna be my approach to figuring this out. So it doesn't always work the whole—see one, do one, teach one thing—because I have to kind of stop and figure things out on my own in between.

One nurse felt that whether or not you get accommodations depends on the kind of job you have: "Well usually the higher up you are, the more likely you are to be able to get accommodations and facilitate the kind of job you want to do." One's position in the organization should not influence whether or not the nurse receives an accommodation.

One nurse with knee pain found ways to compensate using a wheelchair.

I was able to put all my paperwork and all the equipment I needed to carry around with me in the wheelchair and they accused me of using the wheelchair to ride around with instead of walking behind it. I don't sit in a wheelchair, I push it and all my equipment sits in the chair.

This nurse was made to get a walker at her own expense. "I was able to put all my equipment into the walker and push it along with me, if I needed it." Since the law requires that reasonable accommodations be made, they should not be offered only to people high up in the organization or be provided only if the nurse pays for them out of pocket. Both scenarios are unacceptable.

Another nurse with multiple sclerosis had received a letter from her physician outlining for her employer what she could and couldn't do in her job. She was told by her employer that she would get no accommodation or job sharing, nor would a job be created for her. At one point her supervisor held a meeting with her and other staff to specifically discuss how each staff member felt about this nurse having a disability. She felt that the environment became untenable and eventually took an early retirement and obtained disability benefits.

I think it was because toward the end I got a mouth on me and I started making my needs known and maybe people got tired of listening to me.... Nothing was ever mentioned. My physician called me at home and said "I get the impression that they don't want you there anymore" and I said [that] I get the same impression so despite the letter he had written, they didn't offer to work with me to find out anything else, they just kind of took everything like you're going to retire, so just retire . . . I figured that there was so much animosity with the staff I worked with that I thought this is probably for right now the right thing to do, let it rest.

Another nurse who had minimal function in one knee and had to be on crutches for a temporary period of time spoke of the work load she was given after her return to work from surgery.

Once I started trying to get back out onto the floor, it was obvious that I wasn't functioning well, so [the supervisor] started giving me projects [so] that I'd not be assigned to patients that day, but I'd be assigned to, let's say, admissions where it was sedentary, basically paperwork. . . . I was put on light duty so I was restricted for lifting. I had to be doing sedentary work. . . .

Performing desk work that was nonetheless work that was needed to be done was a way of compensating for what the nurse could not then provide in the form of bedside care. She was surprised, however, that the other things that one might consider necessary to doing a desk job were not provided.

I don't know if I'd call it a compensation, but one would think that somebody who isn't able to walk that well would perhaps get a phone so that they could make contact with people that they need to get in touch with. That was something that was never given to me so I still have to get up and walk to get where I need to go to talk to anybody on the unit which is a giant pain, literally and figuratively. It took me 9 months to get my own computer. . . .

Not having a phone and the difficulty getting a computer so she could do her work were ". . . like the biggest slaps in the face. [It's as if they are saying] 'We understand that you're valuable and that you need to do these things but we're not gonna make it easy for you.'"

Another nurse with severe arthritis, especially in the hip, talked of how she compensates for what she cannot do easily:

I might just [need to compensate] when I take blood pressures. I take a different body stance. Where before I could bend over and do it. I can't bend at my waist anymore, I have to bend at my hips. I have to pivot on that hip joint, 'cause the rods don't bend. My biggest difficulty is looking for IVs that are hanging. I have to step back to see up. . . . I can't turn my hips sideways so if I'm looking down—we have five beds in a row—if I'm down at number one, I have to really kind of turn my whole body to look and make sure number five is okay. . . . I have a walker in the car if I have to walk long distances. . . . Just in case I need it. . . . I still say [that] except for my walking ability, I could still do the ER. You know, give me an electric wheelchair and I'll do it that way instead. . . . I'd have to make accommodations. . . .

This nurse was pleased with her job and how well she was treated. Regarding her boss, she said: "She's been wonderful, just wonderful. And all they do is sing my praise. . . . They said 'We are so glad we took a chance and went with you.'"

A nurse who worked both as a school nurse and as a health counselor and who wore hearing aids said:

I'm finding it more difficult in meetings to comprehend everything that is being said and I do everything I can to compensate like sit up close, make sure my hearing aids are [working]. I have digital hearing aids. . . . I do tell people I'm hard of hearing, please look at me when you talk but . . . I gotta take blood pressures . . . and do monthly assessments [so] I have to take my hearing aids out to do blood pressures . . . and then I have to stop and put them back in to be able to talk with [patients] and get updated health history from them.

When asked how others respond to her requests, she answered:

They will attend to it but then they tend to forget unless I keep reminding them. . . . I hope that things are in writing after, so I could review what I understand to clarify so . . . in team meetings if we're discussing children or whatever, I get the written part after[ward] which is helpful . . . [to]make sure I'm understanding everything that's said.

Regarding the use of the phone she stated that as long as she could turn the volume up on the ear piece, she was able to hear without special devices. This nurse is also diabetic and has had to be her own advocate regarding the need to eat at certain times.

Your heart's pounding, you're sweating and you can't comprehend what people are telling you, so I have to say . . . I'm a diabetic, I need to go eat something or I need to stop right now, which can cause difficulty when you're in the middle of doing something really important or in the middle of a crisis or something.

This nurse described the support of a colleague that was instrumental in being able to remain in nursing despite a disability.

> Having support.... [like] another nurse who was hearing impaired she helped me [by saying] why don't you go to the Bureau of Rehab [and get financial help with hearing aids]. No one tells you what kinds of things are out there and I've gone online and everything is expensive.... [It's hard to find out] what's out there to help you to do your job or what the employer is required to provide for you to do your specific job.

This nurse asked her employers if a flashing light might accompany a telephone buzzer that she found to be very faint as the phone did not actually ring. She was told that this accommodation would be too expensive. When she has tried to tell people she is hard of hearing, especially when people walk up behind her and she doesn't know they are talking to her, people don't take her seriously.

> It makes it very difficult... they'll be saying excuse me and I don't even hear them. All of a sudden they'll pat me on the shoulder.... [I say] Oh, I'm sorry, I'm hard of hearing and they laugh and I'm like *no*, I'm serious, I'm hard of hearing.... People joke about that stuff. I get people [who] joke to me all the time ... which is very difficult. I don't think they mean to hurt you but they'll [say] turn your hearing aids up or they'll make movements to me with their fingers like they're talking to me in sign language. It's very difficult especially when you're a professional and you have to get treated that way.

One nurse working in the operating room talked about how staff reacted when it became obvious that he was having trouble walking:

> Well most of the staff were very caring and did what they could to help me ... everybody was very kind, cordial, and supportive, but obviously when it got to the point where I was having to use two canes to get around they would do things like push the patients down the hall for me which was considerate. Fortuitously, having to do a lot of things that are done in floor nursing where you roll patients and lift patients and so forth, these were not in my role....

This nurse had to make some compensations when he developed a problem with mobility.

> For example, pushing a patient from the pre-op back to surgery and helping to roll patients from a gurney onto an operating room table [was difficult].... It was always my habit to carry small

pediatric [patients] like under 3 years [old] back in my arms and also take them in my arms from surgery to recovery but once I developed this mobility problem, I couldn't do that anymore and I had to put the patient on a gurney and walk beside.

Interestingly, this nurse found other nurses to be supportive but the surgeons he worked with tended not to be so supportive. Interestingly the culture from which the surgeons came seemed to influence how they treated him.

Nursing was supportive. Some of the surgeons were absolutely not supportive and as a matter of fact took it as an opportunity to throw barbs and digs: "We can do better" and that sort of thing. . . . "Get a nondisabled person." . . . American-born surgeons were supportive and caring and [said] "Hey, take your time, do what you gotta do." The attitude was considerably different.

He also found there to be gender differences regarding how nurses treat each other:

Women, ladies tend to be far harder on their colleagues, you've heard the term "nursing eats its young." I don't know why that is but women tend to be much harder on each other than men do. I think when it comes to minor differences like this and so forth. I don't know if that's a biased observation but it's an observation. . . . I sat on the board of nursing for awhile and the tales of heroism by nursing that came across that desk everyday were an inspiration. I mean nurses are heroes, but they can be real hard on each other.

A nurse summed things up:

You know the world is different today, the working world is different today. . . . I'm old enough that I've worked the many years that I've seen changes and I think it's a pretty tough world out there.

SOLUTIONS

Clearly, nurses with disabilities just like everyone else, experience varying interactions with colleagues, patients, and clients. Nurses with disabilities are often supported, more frequently viewed askance, and sometimes teased. They are made to prove themselves that much more than others are because they may need to do things differently and others are likely to assume that any way that is different could not possibly be correct.

Nurse educators and leaders set the tone for how nursing students who become new nurses and how working nurses perceive and treat nurses with disabilities. Every nurse will age and with age often comes debility. If older nurses continue to stay at work, they too will experience the need to make compensations and receive accommodations. Consequently, all nurses should be sympathetic to their colleagues who may need assistance due to disability or chronic illness that may be unrelated to age. Nursing must work to build a culture of appreciation for one another and model that behavior to others.

REFERENCES

Neal-Boylan, L. (2012). An exploration and comparison of the worklife experiences of registered nurses and physicians with permanent physical and/or sensory disabilities. *Rehabilitation Nursing, 37*(1), 3–10.

Neal-Boylan, L., Hopkins, A., Skeete, R., Hartmann, S. B., Iezzoni, L. I., & Nunez-Smith, M. (2012). The career trajectories of health care professionals practicing with permanent disabilities. *Academic Medicine, 87*(2), 172–78.

BIBLIOGRAPHY

Guillett, S. E., Neal-Boylan, L. J., & Lathrop, R. (2007). Ready, willing, and disabled. *American Nurse Today, 2*(8), 30–32.

Neal-Boylan, L., Fennie, K., & Baldauf-Wagner, S. (2011). Nurses with sensory disabilities: Their perceptions and characteristics. *Rehabilitation Nursing, 36*(1), 25–31.

Neal-Boylan, L., & Guillett, S. E. (2008a). Registered nurses with physical disabilities. *Journal of Nursing Administration, 38*(1), 1–3.

Neal-Boylan, L., & Guillett, S. E. (2008b). Work experiences of RNs with physical disabilities. *Rehabilitation Nursing, 33*(2), 67–72.

Neal-Boylan, L. J., & Guillett, S. E. (2008c). Nurses with disabilities: Can changing our educational system keep them in nursing? *Nurse Educator, 33*(4), 1–4.

7

Nurse Heroics

Roger, a 50-year-old registered nurse with chronic back pain, worked in an outpatient pediatric clinic. It was a fast-paced environment and Roger was the only RN. Roger supervised nurse's aides and licensed practical nurses as they assisted three physicians and three nurse practitioners to care for pediatric patients with acute and chronic illnesses and injuries. Roger knew his job well and was very good at delegating responsibility but he was well aware that there were many things that only an RN, by law, could do. He also enjoyed his patients and their families and felt that it was important to take the time to educate them about their child's condition before they left the clinic. Many of the patients and families were indigent and he knew that they often needed help beyond the medical complaint that brought them into the clinic. While the clinic was open and patients were being seen, Roger would focus his time on assisting the providers and teaching patients. He would save his administrative work for after hours and weekends. He also made time to periodically educate his staff on the latest in pediatric nursing and care. He felt it important to help them maintain their expertise. He also felt a responsibility to keep his staff happy at work so they could pass on that feeling to their patients and make children and families feel as comfortable as possible while in the clinic. Consequently, Roger often made time after hours to listen to his staff and their concerns about their lives. It was often quite late when Roger arrived home and turned his attention to his partner and his home. He often felt fatigued and in pain. He did not mention his own hardships to anyone at work because he believed that, as a nurse, he was only doing his job and that his own health concerns counted little against the needs of his patients and staff.

Nurses with disabilities talk about "nurse heroics." They use the term to describe all of the things nurses do including working overtime, working when ill, and most interestingly, the expectation in the profession that nurses never stop being nurses. During research interviews, this phenomenon came up frequently and is an important theme regarding the experience of being a nurse with a disability. As one nurse with rheumatoid arthritis says regarding when she had an episode of acute illness "But I didn't tell anyone there. . . . I thought, it's better to just buck up and not say anything."

There appears to be a scarcity of literature regarding nurse heroics unrelated to the response to a crisis, war, or military duty. One may find individual stories about nurses who have worked above and beyond the call of duty, but research regarding this topic is hard to find. However, there is literature that discusses nurse burnout, fatigue, and stress, and how these impact nursing work. This chapter will discuss the idea of nurse heroics with regard to how nurses, in general, and nurses with disabilities in particular feel that they must push themselves beyond what might otherwise seem reasonable.

WHAT IS MEANT BY "NURSE HEROICS?"

In the literature, the term refers to nursing heroes or to nurses who respond to a crisis. However, in the research regarding nurses with disabilities, nurses coined the term to mean that they are expected to work through their pain and fatigue and to not complain (Box 7.1). Nurses with disabilities, by and large, found that they were not given any additional leeway in the expectations of the work just because they had a disability. Even if others offered verbal understanding, when it came to asking to trade shifts or to not have to float to another unit because of issues related to pain or fatigue, the nurses with disabilities were most frequently viewed as slackers.

Box 7.1 Characteristics of Nurse Heroics

Working overtime
Working on vacation days
Changing shifts often
Missing meal breaks
Missing coffee breaks
Floating to other units frequently
Working more hours than required by the shift
Working despite pain, illness, or overwhelming fatigue
Uncomplaining

Nurses, in general, often make a choice to do more than what might reasonably be expected of them because they see themselves as totally devoted to the patient and their colleagues and they derive satisfaction from being viewed by patients, colleagues, and administrators as giving everything they have to the profession. Often, nurses genuinely get attached to patients and families and want to "be there" for them in ways that go beyond standard patient care. Many nurses visit their patients when they are off duty just to check on them and attend funerals of patients they took care of. The latter are choices the nurse makes so they might not view them as heroic, but when the choice is made for the nurse regarding how much they should work or in what ways they should work, then that may be perceived as beyond what should be expected. As one nurse with a disability put it:

> Instead of using my hands to lift a patient, I'll . . . lift a leg so I can see a wound, and I'll use a sheet to pull up so I don't have to use my fingers and I'll try to maneuver that way. . . . I can have strength to a point so there are a lot of times I push myself, I may have a lot of pain later. Obviously if I'm in a client's home and I need to do something, I'm gonna do it and deal with what happens to me afterwards.

Fagerstrom (2006), in a hermeneutical study of nurses, found that putting patients first is an ethical imperative among nurses. Nurses struggle between wanting to provide the best care possible and the external pressures they feel that are not directly related to patient care.

In the study (Fagerstrom, 2006), nurses described optimal nursing care from the nurse's perspective as having the time to attend to patient needs, spiritual as well as physical. External pressures such as working conditions may prevent the nurse from having as much time as he or she would like to have with patients. When the nurse is hurried, only the necessary duties that typically focus on physical care get performed and both nurses and patients find this dissatisfying.

The feeling of not having control over one's time can lead to burnout and errors. Additionally, when nurses are faced with heavy workloads, they have difficulty coping and fear that they will make mistakes. Chaotic times also serve to wear down collegial relationships and relationships with patients' families (Fagerstrom, 2006) because there is not enough time to cultivate these relationships.

Despite this, the nurses in the study (Fagerstrom, 2006) considered the chaotic times to be inevitable consequences of caring for sick patients. They viewed being able to spend quality time with patients despite the tasks needed to keep the unit running smoothly as optimal. The nurses saw the patients as having the inherent right to receive quality nursing care and that this right is paramount to all else. The nurse should provide the care that the patient needs.

When nurses have some flexibility to prioritize and plan care as they see fit while meeting the needs of the patient, they feel more control over situations and that there is harmony to the situations. Nurses are constantly struggling between what they want to see happen and what can be done but are realistic in the sense that they recognize that demanding work is inherent in nursing. A balance between doing the demanding work and still having time to meet the holistic needs of patients makes their work significant (Fagerstrom, 2006).

The ethical imperative of wanting to provide patients with the best possible care leads to the struggle between "being a good nurse" and wanting to provide good care and "not being a good nurse" because the work is hampered by external conditions such as those required by the organization or facility (Fagerstrom, 2006, p. 630). Perhaps it is this struggle that subconsciously leads nurses to sacrifice their own time and well-being in service to their patients.

The scarcity of literature about the phenomenon of nurses making each other feel as if they must work above and beyond all of the time may be because nurses themselves don't typically see this as anything unusual. Nurses have been conditioned to put the patient first and rightly so, but in doing so, the activities and demands that consume so much of their time and that are not related to direct patient care may be lumped together with what nurses perceive to be patient care. In other words, nurses may take for granted that working varying shifts, forgoing breaks and mealtimes, and working when they are supposed to be off demonstrate their commitment to patient care even if those things aren't directly related to the care of the patient. This may explain why nurses may not ask for help to move heavy patients and consequently hurt their backs. The patient needs to be moved or turned or lifted and consequently the nurse performs that action, often not thinking or only thinking later about the consequences to his or her own person.

If Fagerstrom's (2006) findings are true for nurses in general, then it may be unfair to hold supervisors or managers responsible for "nurse heroics" when it is nurses ourselves who make the sacrifices we feel we need to make for our patients. Although, as the researcher suggests, if managers understand the conflict within nurses regarding wanting to provide quality nursing care but also needing to meet external demands, then perhaps careful staff scheduling can help. She also suggests that nurse managers examine the external conditions that may contribute to chaotic work situations and try to decrease their impact.

Nurse educators are certainly in a position to change this cultural aspect of nursing by teaching students that they must take care of themselves in order to be able to take care of their patients. Nursing students should be made to understand that while the patient comes first, their own health is not expendable and that they have value to the organization and must therefore be rested when they come to work so they can handle crises and chaotic situations. This can only help if nurse managers support this cultural change in the workplace. Otherwise, new graduates may be set up to fail if they are groomed to advocate for themselves in the workplace and they are made to feel that they are not team players.

A recent class of graduate nursing students, who were varied based on how long they had been registered nurses, described feeling wary and reluctant to say no when asked by their supervisors to come in on their days off or to work late even when they wanted or needed to be home. They described getting the distinct impression that they would not be viewed as team players or as one of "them" if they weren't willing to drop everything to work longer, work harder, or work on a day they would have been off. Interestingly, the newer nurses were very hesitant and did not typically speak up to managers about their personal plans or need to decline. They did what was asked of them. The more experienced nurses, by and large, had found ways to protect their personal time without being viewed as slacking but they were careful to accept additional work in order to "earn" their time off. In other words, they recognized that sacrifices still had to be made in order to be viewed as a good worker and team player. No one can totally avoid coming in when they are supposed to be off or not staying and working overtime without some backlash. When asked if peers or supervisors told her she was not being a team player, one nurse with a disability said:

> I think I policed myself on that. . . . I can think of one person in particular who would occasionally take mental health days to try to get some time for herself and she was considered to be unreliable and . . . you [would] get that sort of back talk about her. . . . I [can] think of other people, but she was a peer in the sense that she was another clinician and so that [was] particularly relevant to what I would think would happen if I were to do the same thing.

Nurses are in the business of counseling patients and they know about reducing stress and the importance of sleep, rest, and relaxation. Yet here is another example in which nurses ask patients to do what they say, not what they do. To take a "mental health day" even when the nurse has earned time and is entitled to take days off is often viewed as letting the rest of the staff down and not pulling one's weight. This becomes even more pronounced for nurses with disabilities as they frequently need help to do their work and are often hampered by fatigue and pain.

> I think there's definitely some heroism involved in the whole nursing concept . . . it's the irony of you tell your patients to do all these good things to take care of themselves but you expect that you don't have to worry, that it doesn't apply to you as far as taking time for yourself and not over committing and not allowing your job to overtax you and all those things you try to tell people. Yeah, I've seen a lot with nursing that we're expected to go above and beyond because it's a heroic kind of job. (Neal-Boylan & Guillett, 2008a)

A TRADITION OF SELF-SACRIFICE

The idea that nurses should work long and hard is not new, perhaps it is as old as nursing itself. Florence Nightingale set the standard for how nurses should present themselves and carry out their duties and proscribed that their behavior should be beyond reproach. Their focus was to, at all times, protect and advocate for the patient. It is interesting to note that in her chapter "Petty management" in *Notes on Nursing: What It Is and What It Is Not* (http://digital.library.upenn.edu/women/nightingale/nursing/nursing.html#III), she cautions the nurse to not overwork herself but to take needed breaks and to explain to the patient that this is necessary to the nurse's health and well-being.

> All the results of good nursing, as detailed in these notes, may be spoiled or utterly negatived by one defect, viz.: in petty management, or in other words, by not knowing how to manage that what you do when you are there, shall be done when you are not there. The most devoted friend or nurse cannot be always *there*. Nor is it desirable that she should. And she may give up her health, all her other duties, and yet, for want of a little management, be not one-half so efficient as another who is not one-half so devoted, but who has this art of multiplying herself—that is to say, the patient of the first will not really be so well cared for, as the patient of the second.
>
> But it is possible to press upon her to think for herself: Now what does happen during my absence? I am obliged to be away on Tuesday. But fresh air, or punctuality is not less important to my patient on Tuesday than it was on Monday. Or: At 10 p.m. I am never with my patient; but quiet is of no less consequence to him at 10 than it was at 5 minutes to 10.
>
> Curious as it may seem, this very obvious consideration occurs comparatively to few, or, if it does occur, it is only to cause

the devoted friend or nurse to be absent fewer hours or fewer minutes from her patient—not to arrange so as that no minute and no hour shall be for her patient without the essentials of her nursing.

At all events, one may safely say, a nurse cannot be with the patient, open the door, eat her meals, take a message, all at one and the same time. Nevertheless the person in charge never seems to look the impossibility in the face. (p. 35)

Nightingale essentially gives nurses permission and actually requests of them that they take care of themselves and rely on their qualified colleagues to cover for them when they need to be away from the patient. Needing to take care of oneself does not make the nurse less efficient or less of a good nurse.

"The person in charge" (p. 35) as Nightingale puts it, becomes the obstacle, according to many nurses, and everyone else not wanting to appear as slackers buys into this notion that nursing is completely selfless and that nurses should be available at all times. It is interesting that this perception of nurses regarding being a good nurse has not seemed to change since Nightingale's time.

The author's grandmother graduated nursing school in 1920 and spoke of picketing with other nurses to be able to work five, 8-hour days per week. She and her colleagues were working six, 12-hour days per week. When she heard about modern nurses wanting to work 12 hour shifts she was amazed and appalled. Even when it was explained that the nurse would work three, 12-hour days each week, the author's grandmother said that this did not help to lessen the work expectations of the nurse but perhaps make them worse. Nurses today often claim that they work harder than nurses have in the past. Historically, nurses did not have all of the high technology equipment we have now nor were they given the same degree of responsibility. However, the author's grandmother would respond to this by saying that nurses, in her day, had the responsibility for an entire hospital floor from the time they were students and that they also had to sterilize equipment that was not disposable at that time. In short, nurses from previous generations can make an excellent case for having worked just as hard, if not harder than nurses today.

The author's mother is also a nurse and graduated from nursing school in 1953. She, like so many other diploma school graduates, spoke of being in charge of the hospital while a student, working long shifts, and also attending classes full time. The nurses lived in dormitories that were strictly monitored so the author's father and other young men who were inclined to visit the student nurses had to be chaperoned while the couples visited in the visiting room. Not only were the student nurses' school work and clinical practica closely supervised with high expectations for performance considered the norm, but their private lives were closely monitored as well. It was felt that the image of the nurse as chaste, sound of body and mind, and focused on providing quality nursing care must not be tainted by one's social activities.

One nurse with a disability spoke about this in her organization.

> I guess it was sort of the general work ethic of the organization which was that if you were asked to do more, you did more. A lot of the sort of upper management people worked way more hours than the forty hours and so that was sort of the expectation, you do whatever they need you to do, which is . . . a common expectation of a lot of workplaces these days. (Neal-Boylan & Guillett, 2008a, 2008b)

The literature speaks of the long work hours and lack of committed breaks and rest times for nurses despite the fact that nurses comprise such a large portion of the health care workers in the country (Witkoski & Dickson, 2010). Nurses forego their breaks so they can take care of their patients and it is an expectation that they will do so while other professions that also have to be concerned about safety, such as pilots and professional drivers, are limited in the hours they can work.

There are no standardized limitations on nurse work hours (Bureau of Labor Statistics, 2009; Witkoski & Dickson, 2010) despite the fact that musculoskeletal problems have been found to be related to long work hours and the physical requirements of nursing (Trinkoff, Le, Geiger-Brown, Lipscomb, & Lang, 2006). One nurse educator said:

> My therapist . . . kept saying to me you really need to rest more and take more time for yourself and I agree with her and I try to do that but I'm just a Type A and it's in my blood. I don't know how to do less than I'm doing.

Nurses may not be paid for a meal break and yet they frequently work during their meal break (Witkoski & Dickson, 2010). To be working during their meal break and to not receive compensation implies that it is a given that nurses must take care of patients first and forego their own needs for food and rest. In conversation with each other about taking a meal or a coffee break, nurses often react with sarcastic laughter because it is often a joke that the nurse will get an opportunity to take a break. Nurses with diabetes mellitus, for instance, who were interviewed commented that even with their physiological need to have scheduled mealtimes, it was not uncommon for them to have to insist that they leave the floor to eat.

Frequently, they waited until they could not possibly wait any longer to make it known that they had to get food immediately. Sometimes it has been necessary for diabetic nurses to specifically ask other nurses to cover for them so they could leave. Ideally, this should already happen and not just for diabetic nurses but for all nurses as everyone needs food and time to reenergize.

The counter argument, in this case and so often in any discussion of workload, is the lack of staff and that staff is insufficient to cover breaks and days off. However, many nurses respond that as long as nurses are willing to be "heroic" and not demand that they take scheduled breaks at the time they are scheduled, then administrators will not feel compelled to spend the money to hire more staff.

A recent study of more than 2,000 nurses in 11 countries found that the majority felt that they had a more difficult workload than 5 years previous. Nurses felt that they worked harder than they used to and 46% of the nurses in the United States who participated in the study reported that "nursing as a career [is] worse today than it was 5 years ago" (DeCola & Riggins, 2010, p. 336). Nurses cited time constraints regarding patient care and responded that more time providing patient care to individual patients would make a significant difference in the health of patients (DeCola & Riggins, 2010).

Burnout (Box 7.2) is a common problem among nurses and can be precipitated by demanding work expectations (Hayes & Bonner, 2010). Burnout is another issue that is becoming more prevalent in the literature as nurses leave nursing to pursue other careers or positions outside of inpatient care. People who are burned out tend to be exhausted. This exhaustion can be manifested by a feeling of inability to continue to give, by distancing oneself from relationships, and by beginning to feel incompetent or cynical (Maslach, 2001, 2009; Pereira, Fonseca, & Carvalho, 2011).

Box 7.2   Characteristics of Burnout

- "Prolonged response to chronic interpersonal stressors on the job" (Maslach, 2009, p. 498; Maslach & Jackson, 1981)
- *Exhaustion:* "feelings of being overextended and depleted of one's emotional and physical resources" (Maslach, 2009, p. 498)
- *Cynicism or depersonalization:* "negative, callous or excessively detached response to various aspects of the job" (Maslach, 2009, p. 498)
- *Inefficacy (reduced accomplishment):* "feelings of incompetence and a lack of achievement and productivity in work"(Maslach, 2009, p. 498)

One who is experiencing burnout may feel more vulnerable and develop physical symptoms of illness (Pereira et al., 2011) and stress-induced illness (Maslach, 2009). Burnout has been correlated with job dissatisfaction, absenteeism, and leaving the job (Maslach, 2009). A recent study by Maslach (who has done a lot of the research on burnout) found that it is possible to identify people who are inclined to burnout. The study found that people who perceived unfairness toward them in the workplace were more likely to develop signs of burnout as opposed to those who might display exhaustion or cynicism but did not perceive unfairness. An aspect of the perception of unfairness was job inequity and the perception that the wrongs done to the person will not be righted by administrators. The researcher suggests that individualized intervention might prevent burnout. Counseling or additional job training are proposed as examples (Maslach, 2009).

This research has interesting implications for nurses with disabilities. Since research thus far on this population has showed a high risk of leaving the nursing profession, it is fair to say that burnout may be a potential reason. If administrators are aware that burnout occurs because of perceived injustices—being treated differently because of having a disability—then, perhaps they can take proactive steps to prevent a perception of unfairness by giving nurses with disabilities the chances they need to demonstrate their ability to perform the job.

Burnout can occur when the expectations of the nurse regarding his or her role and the support the nurse receives in that role by the organization are not congruent. Gradually, the nurse feels worn down and cannot continue at the previous pace (Sabo, 2006). Burnout can happen to any nurse but if one figures that the nurse with a disability is already starting from a point of fatigue and possibly pain, as well as a need to compensate for what he or she may not be able to do in the usual way, than it seems logical that the nurse with a disability who is not given the opportunity to rest or take breaks might burnout more quickly.

The literature also talks about hardiness (Box 7.3) and how that personal characteristic may help prevent exhaustion, which can lead to burnout. Hardiness is considered to be a combination of 3 factors: Feeling committed, feeling in control, and a perception of change as something

Box 7.3   Characteristics of Hardiness

- A sense of commitment
- A perception of control
- The ability to view change as a challenge

challenging (Bryant, 1994; Schwab, 1996). A nurse with this characteristic perceives stress as a positive thing and is able to use his or her other personality resources to avoid illness during times of stress.

This book has included some stories from nurses who took pride in being able to meet the challenges of nursing work despite having a disability and who felt they would stay in nursing even if that meant going from job to job to find something that they could do or that would provide the accommodations they needed. As one nurse said:

> I think I have kind of a high tolerance for pain because I really do power through it. . . . Which is why I continue to do movement even though . . . it hurts. . . . I'm not willing to just sit back and say "Okay, I just can't do this."

More often, however, the stories from nurses with disabilities have included the need to take whatever was offered and to accept the jobs that were given because they could not expect anything else nor did they feel necessarily entitled to anything else.

The commitment of the nurses with disabilities who were interviewed cannot be in doubt as the nurses who agreed to be interviewed and surveyed said that they did so because they want the system to change so they can stay in nursing and do what they love. It is the feeling of control and the perception of changes wrought by having a disability as positive challenges that may be lacking in many of the nurses studied. That may also depend on how long they had been working with a disability, their type of disability, and the type of nursing work they were doing.

Nurses with disabilities who were actively working (the fourth study described in Chapter 1) had chosen jobs, mostly because of their disabilities, that they felt they could do and still remain in nursing. These nurses had actively sought these jobs. In some cases, nurses who were working in jobs in which having a disability was becoming a problem were actively looking for other jobs. Perhaps this intentional search for jobs they could do with their disabilities in mind speaks to their sense of control. Many nurses interviewed for the previous studies had left nursing and despaired because they felt there were no jobs they could do. However, those that were working, and were happy in their jobs, were either making their situations accommodate them or were actively seeking jobs that could accommodate their needs. One might surmise that the nurses with disabilities who were *happily* working had more of a sense of control than the nurses with disabilities who were not working in nursing. Again, this is a gross generalization as age, type of disability, and other factors inevitably play roles in the choices nurses make, but it is worth considering as is this concept of viewing change as a positive challenge.

ACHIEVING A BALANCE

The ability to balance work and home life is another factor to consider when examining the impact of nurse heroics. Nurses may feel guilty when they don't think they have done enough at work and the same way about their home life when they don't have enough time to do what they want to do at home. Consistently sacrificing ourselves for our patients may ultimately lead to feeling exhausted and burned out. Achieving a balance in which the nurse can feel good about leaving when the shift is done or taking a vacation is vital to preventing self-neglect. It is important to determine when being a perfectionist is really necessary and when one has done enough to satisfy the requirement without jeopardizing anyone's well-being or quality of care. It may be necessary to cut corners on things that are less important so nurses have the energy and wherewithal to do the important things (Chittenden & Ritchie, 2011).

A nurse with rheumatoid arthritis said:

> I think the other thing which plays a role is [that] I'm a person who holds very high expectations for myself, so if I'm not meeting my own expectations I feel bad and I kind of feel like everybody around me should be disappointed I'm not meeting the expectations when I actually may be setting my own expectations too high . . .

It is natural and common to think that others are able to do it all while we cannot and that we must push ourselves harder and do better or work longer. However, in reality, others may be struggling with the same doubts (Chittenden & Ritchie, 2011). Perhaps if nurses talked about this issue more openly in their own facilities and organizations and everyone openly admitted to feeling the need for balance, there would be less behind the back snickering and animosity if someone takes a mental health break with days they've earned.

An internal locus of control, meaning the ability to take responsibility for what happens to us rather than laying blame on others, can help us cope under stress (Chittenden & Ritchie, 2011; Kobasa, 1979). However, the down side of always feeling an internal locus of control is that we constantly blame ourselves for not being able to do everything all of the time and then feel guilty or insecure as a result (Chittenden & Ritchie, 2011). Nurses with disabilities who leave nursing may feel that it is completely their responsibility to be able to do everything their colleagues can do and in the same way. Rather than demanding their legal right to reasonable accommodation or disability or sick leave or seeking other jobs that may be a better fit, they may feel that it is better to leave the profession so others do not feel responsible for them or for their work experiences.

Patients may take for granted that nurses sacrifice their own needs to care for their patients. This may be why nurses are among the most trusted professionals. Interestingly, there is little in the literature about the patient's image of nursing other than with regard to which uniforms they wear or how the media portrays them. There seems little to no discussion about whether patients view the nurse as working too hard. The "angel of mercy" image and the "lady with the lamp" image seem the most common positive images of nursing until someone requires the services of a nurse and develops an appreciation for what nurses do and how much they need to know. At that point, patients often remark on how hard nurses work and on how much having an attentive and capable nurse meant to them.

NURSES WITH DISABILITIES AND HEROICS

Nurses with disabilities described how they viewed "nurse heroics" and how they were clearly not seen as exempt, in most cases, from being heroic. Nurse heroics was one of the major themes that came out of the original study and was echoed in the research that followed. The nurses with disabilities spoke of heroics in the context of having a disability and having to still fit the image of the nurse as the person who never stopped working for fear of failing the patient and colleagues.

Nurses with disabilities often held themselves to the same high heroic standard. Many nurses who felt that they could not maintain a high standard of heroics—work long hours, be willing to work any shift, etc.—left nursing or their current job for another one that was less demanding. As one nurse put it: "I think the choices I made were my own but they were made from the baseline that I had to keep up with everything." Another nurse said: "And I'm the type of person that I give it 200 percent. And I couldn't manage that with them (that facility)." These nurses made choices that eventually involved leaving their nursing positions.

The need to keep up with the demands of nursing and patient care seems to be so strong that nurses in general, and nurses with disabilities in particular, are willing to damage and jeopardize their own health to do so. A nurse who worked in the hospital said:

> I think my surgeon was the one that basically told me that the more walking I did and the more pain I tried to work through, the more I would damage my joints and increase the arthritis, and he said on down the road you might be paying for what you're doing right now trying to stay on your feet all day.

This nurse did continue to work but eventually got a nursing job in a non-hospital setting. Nurses are supposed to pretend to be superhuman and to not have pain or discomfort or even a bad day. A recent study (Wood & Marshall, 2010) explored the attitude of nurse leaders toward nurses with disabilities. All of the nurse leaders surveyed worked in hospitals and most of them reported having worked with a nurse with a disability. A large percentage (41%) of the nurse leaders said that they had "high to severe concerns" (p. 184) about nurses with disabilities and work performance. There was also "high to severe" (p. 184) concern regarding the need of nurses with disabilities to leave work for doctor's appointments. This confirms that there seems to be an assumption that nurses with disabilities cannot pull their own weight, let alone meet the "heroic" demands that all nurses must meet in day-to-day work. Interestingly, this particular study also showed that nurse leaders who had had experience with nurses with disabilities were more likely to be willing to work with them again, indicating that while assumptions are made, they may not bear fruit and that nurses with disabilities, in actuality, may not have any more problems with work performance and absenteeism than do other nurses. The problem is getting past the assumptions so that nurses with disabilities are given a fair chance to demonstrate their capabilities.

One nurse with a disability who was interviewed said:

> My experience in . . . talking with other people in the field or working with other people in the field [is that] it's [the] same sorta expectation to mask or to go past whatever physical limitations you might have, to not bring that to the table, to not say "I really need you to modify something." . . . I think there is that expectation you are the strong person, you're the nurse, you're the caretaker, not the one that other people are supposed to be taking care of and that's another piece of nursing, about what you'll do for your patients, but not for yourself. You're the caretaker. . . . I think there might be certain things that people have learned . . . physical conditions that people have some understanding about. I think diabetes is pretty well known in the culture and pretty well known as far as what diabetes is and what the physical limitations are or what the expectations are. . . . You might be able to put it out there and say . . . I need to eat three times a day . . . and there might be some allowance around that. . . . In nursing, I would think that . . . we're the ones with the knowledge of health care and that we might see a wide range of things that other people don't understand that we might understand better.

It does seem fair to assume that nurses because of our knowledge base would understand the need for other nurses with chronic illnesses or disabilities to need modifications or accommodations in their work but this doesn't seem to happen in actual practice.

Concern for one's colleagues who often have to increase their workload because the nurse with a disability is out sick or at a medical appointment can be the impetus for "pushing through" and working despite pain. One does not want to be viewed by one's colleagues, let alone the supervisor, as having excuses to miss work, no matter how legitimate. One nurse with rheumatoid arthritis said:

> I actually pushed myself and worked a lot. I was in pain a lot and pushed myself 'cause I didn't wanna call out. . . . Many days, I went to work in pain and just sort of pushed through which I don't think is the healthiest thing to do. I would go upstairs one step at a time . . .

If this nurse and others like her are made to feel that they must keep pushing hard despite pain and fatigue, they are likely to reach a point of no return and be unable to continue to work in that setting or, perhaps in nursing. They are likely to achieve exhaustion and burnout more quickly than are other nurses.

Ultimately, the profession loses out because a nurse who might have been valuable for her or his expertise and skills is unable to sustain the heavy workload or the demands of work. Nurse are enculturated to believe that they must not fail their patients or their peers. The author has been told that soldiers frequently feel this way in battle, that "no man is left behind" and that the soldier (or other military service person) in combat sees their primary motivation as supporting his or her comrades and that that becomes their reason for working hard and having high expectations of themselves. This "band of brothers" mentality is not so dissimilar from nursing which (prior to the inculcation of men into the profession) had often been described as a sisterhood in which each woman was empowered by the strength of the bonds with the other women. It is not only nurses with disabilities who push beyond their endurance but nurses in general, tend to feel the need to do this. As one nurse with disabilities said:

> One of the [nurses] used to carry . . . all these charts which I thought was ridiculous. She'd be hauling these charts . . . like 2 pounds of charts . . . with her arms. . . . Then the other nurse who was training me, she had been there a long time, well established. . . . She just ran for everything. She just ran. . . . Sometimes you have to but this is not the emergency room.

This nurse was pointing out that even though she did not work in the emergency department where a reasonable expectation of the job is to move quickly to save lives, her colleagues were running and carrying heavy charts. The latter has become less prevalent with the advent of electronic health records but the principle is the same.

Fletcher (2007) conducted a literature review regarding the public images of nursing and the image nurses have of themselves and the profession. She found that nurses have traditionally been viewed as subservient to men (physicians) and that "the poor nurse is uncaring, incompetent and demonstrates a lack of vocation or calling to nursing" (Fletcher, 2007, p. 209). Her literature review, however, found that nurses' images of themselves included an emphasis on the ability to think critically and be competent clinically. Nurses demonstrate similar behavior to that found in oppressed groups and this explains their tendencies to fight with each other and to be generally nonsupportive of one another. Fletcher concludes that nursing's self-image is closely tied to the issues and problems of the profession itself and to society, in general. "Nurses can no longer be secretly flattered by the stereotypes of dedication and self-sacrifice" (p. 214).

It is an interesting notion that nurses derive secret satisfaction from being seen as self-sacrificing and yet they otherwise complain that they are being overworked and over tasked. It remains a paradox that nurses want to be valued for their intellectual abilities and knowledge but they seem to be the first to identify and punish the nurse who cannot physically pull his or her weight. This book has demonstrated through the stories of the nurses themselves, that even years of nursing practice and expertise cannot often save a nurse with a disability from condemnation by peers and supervisors. However, nurses with disabilities who are currently working in jobs in which they are happy often have nursing supervisors who have had chronic illnesses or disabilities themselves. These supervisors are more likely to tell nurses with disabilities to take care of themselves, to not overwork and overtire themselves and to make sure they get their breaks and rest.

Interestingly, patients are more supportive to an extent in that they view the nurse with a disability as perhaps having more empathy and understanding toward their own limitations and illness than might a fully functional nurse. Patients want their nurses to be competent and to convey competence and they want them to provide comfort and care for them when they are ill or unwell.

As long as nurses are willing to continue to allow themselves to be called in on their days off, to work extra shifts, to be pushed beyond their endurance, to be made to feel that they are not collegial if they don't sacrifice their own health and quality of life for their work, then others will continue to take advantage of them and expect more than can be reasonably given. It reminds one of the emperor's new clothes story by Hans Christian Andersen. Everyone is afraid to anger the emperor by pointing out that he has no clothes on. Nurses are afraid to be seen as slacking so they are reluctant to stand up for themselves and when they do, their colleagues and supervisors are not likely to support them for fear of also being seen as slacking. Research has found that nurses burn out quickly and that fatigue sometimes overwhelms them, yet they still seem to think that their patients would appreciate them more for being self-sacrificing than for being rested and less apt to make errors. As one nurse with rheumatoid arthritis stated:

> I think a lot of people with disabilities tend to be this way that I think you push yourself so hard that sometimes you don't feel you don't realize the impact it's having on you until something's happened and all of a sudden you're sitting back and it's like how was I surviving, how was I doing that?

Nursing is full of contradictions and has a history of not being able to make up its collective mind about what nursing should be. There is no one unifying philosophy of nursing, there is no set entry level for nursing practice, we continue to invent new degrees that must be earned even if there are no data to support them, and so on. We seem to have two different levels, for lack of a better word, of nursing: the ivory tower academics and researchers, and the bedside nurses. Some nurses do both but nurses often leave clinical practice to move on to academe and/or research. Neither group seems particularly respectful of what the other brings to the profession. If we cannot be united in how we view ourselves, then how can we expect others to view us in a certain way and how can we allow ourselves to be more understanding of each other regarding other issues such as disability?

POTENTIAL SOLUTIONS

Ridding ourselves of this notion of nurse heroics will require buy in and cooperation from all levels of the profession. Some may say that we shouldn't get rid of this idea as it is so closely associated with nursing and inspires trust in the profession by the public. On one hand, it may inspire trust, but viewed another way, patients are constantly hearing one thing from us while we model another. Take the high level of obesity and smoking among nurses. We counsel our patients to eat right and to not smoke and expect them to listen and heed.

Patients aren't always aware of the self-sacrificing nature of nursing because they often only know that a nurse is caring for them in a particular setting but not what else the nurse is doing. Patients who are aware may have an image of how hard nurses work instead of how well nurses think. This perception does not help the image of nurses.

People see fireman running into a burning building and policemen getting killed or wounded in the line of duty. This is also seen as self-sacrificing and rightly so. However, does the public want the firemen or policemen to work when they haven't had any sleep or are in too much pain to get to the burning building fast enough or be able to run after the criminal?

In order to refine this notion so that nurses can still be viewed as trustworthy and strong patient advocates, change must begin with entry level nursing education. It is important for nurse educators to teach nursing students not only the value of critical thinking but to value ourselves and not to take our work for granted. Nursing students need to learn how to continue to improve the image of nursing to the public. They should do this by modeling that they take care of themselves as well as dress professionally and demonstrate a high level of knowledge and skill. Just as nurses educate patients and the public about what nurses do, what we can do for them, and how we differ from physicians and other health care providers, we can educate them about how nurses should be valued for modeling healthful behaviors.

Of course, this assumes that nurse educators themselves will be able to model healthful behaviors. As a nurse educator, this author has observed that nurse educators also work themselves beyond exhaustion even when members of other disciplines in the university community manage to take lunch breaks and avoid working on the weekends. In conversation with a prospective graduate student about which area of nursing she should pursue with a graduate degree, this author was told that the student would never consider being a full time academic because "You all work too hard." This is not meant to imply that academics in other disciplines don't work very hard but nurse academics seem to carry the nurse heroics work ethic into the academic setting by being constantly available to students and by leading students to believe that there is no life outside of the university. In order to change what nursing students learn, nurse educators must role model and practice what they intend to preach about caring for ourselves.

Experienced clinical nurses and nurse administrators also need to set the tone for how nurses should be treated while at work. Nurse narratives throughout this book have demonstrated that both clinical colleagues and supervisors tended to view nurses with disabilities as automatically unable to do the job well and as people who would find excuses for missing work or for not working in the same way as nurses without disabilities. This perception remains despite attempts by nurses with disabilities to compensate for what they may be physically unable to do or to trade work with other nurses so that all of the work that needs to be done can get done. If administrators are going to work more than forty hours a week and perhaps the work simply requires that, they should convey to the clinical staff that that does not necessarily mean that staff is expected to work more than 40 hours per week. Administrators set the tone by labeling what is and is not acceptable. If a nurse cannot come in when she or he is supposed to be off, she or he should not have to come up with some "acceptable" excuse, which typically requires that the nurse or someone in their family is sick or dying. Just needing the day off is not considered acceptable. Events do occur when nurses need to fill in for one another but then shouldn't the nurse who came in on the day off be rewarded with time off soon after so he or she can get the necessary rest?

It is not the intention nor the purpose of this book to discuss the financial and other implications of nurse scheduling but merely to emphasize the point that nurses, regardless of their roles, need to get their own rest, both mentally and physically, in order to be at their best when working. Nurses who have been in nursing a long time may have a hard time changing their mindset to permit themselves and their colleagues to say no when asked to work overtime or to work when they're supposed to be off. The ethic of working till you drop may be so far engrained that experienced nurses may have difficulty allowing themselves or others to think differently. Yet, as nurses age, they are more likely to become slowed in their ability to work and are more likely to have a disability. Increased understanding within the profession is likely to benefit their own circumstances.

Nurse leaders, in general, would do a great service to the profession if they espoused an ethic of hard work tempered by time to rest and recover oneself from the day-to-day aspects of nursing. Not only do nurses do physically demanding work and use a lot of mental energy to make critical decisions, they are also consoling the dying and assisting and advising people in difficult circumstances, in crisis, or at times in their lives when they can only confide in the nurse. The nurse is often the repository of patient anger, grief, disappointment, dissatisfaction, and ignorance. Nurses are expected to handle whatever patients tell them or reveal to them with assurances that the nurse will keep things confidential. Often the nurse cannot share his or her own feelings about a patient situation to enable the nurse to cope with difficult situations. All the more reason why nurses need to help each other achieve a balance of work and rest. Nurse leaders can set the tone by role modeling, and by disseminating the view that it is not only acceptable but desirable that nurses not sacrifice themselves to do the job. Sacrifice shouldn't be necessary if the nurse is well trained and is provided with the proper resources to do the work that needs to be done.

Nurse leaders and administrators should push for getting the necessary resources both in manpower and equipment so that nurses can do the job without physically or emotionally injuring themselves. Remember the nurse in Chapter 6 who couldn't get a proper desk or a handicapped parking space despite her disability? Another nurse spoke of not having access to a computer for a long time even though her work required that she use a computer. These types of occurrences are easily remedied. Having enough staff who are qualified to do the job may not be as easy but should the individual nurse continue to be made to feel guilty if he or she doesn't do extra work when the organization has failed to hire enough staff?

Nursing is likely to continue to have periodic shortages and cannot afford to lose good nurses. The literature is replete with publications about how to retain nurses and raise their level of satisfaction. Recognizing that nurses with disabilities are worth keeping and that they need to be allowed to make compensations as long as they are safe is an important step to keeping them in nursing. If their compensations impinge on other staff by increasing their workload than it is up to nursing administrators and leaders to make the resources available so that everyone can do their work without jeopardizing their own health and well-being.

REFERENCES

Bryant, E. (1994). When the going gets tough. *Canadian Nurse, 90*(2), 36–37, 39.

Bureau of Labor Statistics. (2009). *Occupational outlook handbook 2001–2012.* Retrieved from www.bls.gov/oco/ocos083.htm

Chittenden, E. H., & Ritchie, C. S. (2011). Work-life balancing: Challenges and strategies. *Journal of Palliative Medicine, 14*(7), 870–874.

DeCola, P. R., & Riggins, P. (2010). Nurses in the workplace: Expectations and needs. *International Nursing Review, 57*, 335–342.

Fagerstrom, L. (2006). The dialectic tension between "being" and "not being" a good nurse. *Nursing Ethics, 13*(6), 622–632.

Fletcher, K. (2007). Image: Changing how women nurses think about themselves. Literature review. *Journal of Advanced Nursing, 58*(3), 207–215.

Hayes, B., Bonner, A. (2010). Job satisfaction, stress, and burnout associated with haemodialysis nursing: A review of the literature. *Journal of Renal Care, 36*(4), 174–179.

Kobasa, S. C. (1979). Stressful life events, personality, and health: An inquiry into hardiness. *Journal Personal Sociological Psychology, 37*, 1–11.

Maslach, C. (2001). What we have learned about burnout and health. *Psychological Health, 16*, 607–611.

Maslach, C. (2009). Early predictors of job burnout and engagement. *Journal of Applied Psychology, 93*(3), 498–512.

Maslach, C., & Jackson, S. E. (1981). The measurement of experienced burnout. *Journal of Occupational Behavior, 2*, 99–113.

Neal-Boylan, L. J., & Guillett, S. E. (2008a). Nurses with disabilities: Can changing our educational system keep them in nursing? *Nurse Educator, 33*(4), 164–167.

Neal-Boylan, L., & Guillett, S. E. (2008b). Registered nurses with physical disabilities. *Journal of Nursing Administration, 38*(1), 1–3.

Nightingale, F. (1860). *Notes on nursing: What it is and what it is not.* Retrieved from http://digital.library.upenn.edu/women/nightingale/nursing/nursing.html#III.

Pereira, S. M., Fonseca, A. M., & Carvalho, A. S. (2011). Burnout in palliative care: A systematic review. *Nursing Ethics, 18*(3), 317–326.

Sabo, B. M. (2006). Compassion fatigue and nursing work: Can we accurately capture the consequences of caring work? *International Journal of Nursing Practice, 12*, 136–142.

Schwab, L. (1996). Individual hardiness and staff satisfaction. *Nursing Economics, 14*(3), 171–173.

Trinkoff, A. M., Le, R., Geiger-Brown, J., Lipscomb, J., & Lang, G. (2006). Longitudinal relationship of work hours, mandatory overtime, and on-call to musculoskeletal problems in nurses. *American Journal of Industrial Medicine, 49*(11), 964–971.

Witkoski, A., & Dickson, V. V. (2010). Hospital staff nurses' work hours, meal periods, and rest breaks. *AAOHN Journal, 58* (11), 489–497.

Wood, D., & Marshall, E. S. (2010). Nurses with disabilities working in hospital settings: Attitudes, concerns, and experiences of nurse leaders. *Journal of Professional Nursing, 26*(3), 182–187.

8
Retaining Nurses With Disabilities

> I just think that there are so many jobs for nurses right now. . . . So, I think that if a nurse really wants to be in nursing we have to be flexible and find something [they] can do in nursing. It may not be what [they] always thought [they] wanted to do but [they] can still be [doing something that gives them] some self-esteem.

This book has sought to increase awareness regarding the experiences of nurses with physical and/or sensory disabilities. In doing so, the goal has been to encourage the nursing profession to face the issue of discrimination against these nurses and to take concrete steps toward eliminating that discrimination. As nurses, we always begin by assessing, then we plan, act, and finally evaluate the consequences of our interventions. We refer to this as the nursing process. It is hoped that this and other publications will provide the assessment data that nurses need to develop a plan for intervening so that we can stem the flow of nurses with disabilities from our ranks. We can only be sure that the interventions we make are effective if we continually and regularly revisit how nurses with disabilities perceive their experiences in nursing and whether they are leaving the profession.

For a variety of reasons, nurses are remaining in the profession until an advanced age, and retired nurses often continue to work in nursing as volunteers (Cocca-Bates & Neal-Boylan, 2011). Naturally, as such nurses age, they are likely to develop chronic illnesses and disabilities. However, it is not only older nurses but nurses of all ages who can have disabilities.

In addition, the profession is known for its chronic shortage of qualified nurses. Consequently, there clearly is a need to face the fact that we should retain nurses with disabilities and try to meet their needs so as to allow them to continue to work in the field. This book has shown how nurses with experience and expertise are leaving nursing because they no longer feel that they fit in. The profession can make several realistic changes to help these nurses feel like they still belong and want to remain in nursing. This chapter discusses some possible solutions for the rapid loss of nurses with disabilities to the profession and how we might retain them and even recruit people with disabilities to fill the ranks. There are likely many more possible solutions that others may devise. It is hoped that those recommended here will only be a jumping off point to many others.

NURSING EDUCATION

> Yes, [education] gives you different opportunities and . . . for me, it opened up many different areas of my life that I didn't even know existed. . . . Instead of being a tense, angry person because I have a disability, I've been able to say OK, in spite of that I can do something else. . . . I have been fortunate. I've had a lot of supportive people, a lot of mentors who have been there at the right time to say [to me], this is not the end of the world.

Several of the nurses who shared their stories for this book went back to school as a direct consequence of having a disability. They viewed this as a way both to increase their employability and to move away from the very physical work that often accompanies bedside care. Getting another degree certainly did not guarantee that these nurses would find a less physical job or would be treated any differently than in their previous work setting. However, some of them did find that having an additional degree was the key to opening new doors for them both intellectually and professionally. Many remarked that they found new interests as a result and were grateful they had an incentive to go back to school. Others saw it as a strictly practical solution to the difficulties they encountered while trying to work in their ideal nursing job. Yet sometimes they found that it was as difficult to be a nurse with a disability going back to school as it was to be a student nurse with a disability. In some cases, student peers and professors were not supportive.

Nurse educators have tremendous influence on nursing students. It is important that within nursing curricula, educators teach about the experience of having a disability, not only for patients but for those caring for patients. People with disabilities are as diverse as any other group that shares only one common feature that sets them apart from those in the "mainstream." We teach nursing students to respect diversity of all kinds and to relate to patients through what has meaning to the patient.

> I feel that the health professions are . . . really uncomfortable around people with disabilities because I think they could say "Oh my, that could be me." For many medical professionals they have to deny what's going on . . . and I don't feel that they see us as being capable. . . . There's not much taught in nursing school or

medical school though there may be more now. I don't see enough job sharing and education and taking a chance on someone.

The lack of *esprit d'corps* has been a growing problem in nursing that is recognized in the literature through studies on lateral violence and nurses "eating their young." It is clear that nurses don't tend to provide support for one another and that consequently nurse educators are finding it necessary to strengthen their emphasis on caring for one another in the curricula. This focus should extend to a discussion about working with older nurses and nurses with disabilities. Students should be encouraged to value all people for what they bring to the table instead of focusing on what might be missing. A student can learn a lot from an experienced nurse and should look beyond the age or infirmity. As a nurse with a disability put it: ". . . because everybody, everybody will at some point have at least a temporary or at some time, a permanent disability where they will have to go through all those physical and psychological changes, learning how to be dependent, with grace."

It might help for nurse educators in schools of nursing to include presentations by older nurses and nurses with disabilities in which they share their perceptions of their experiences. New nurses often see only their own lack of status and worry that they will be poorly treated as the "new kids on the block." This is a realistic fear but perhaps one that might enable them to empathize with other nurses who aren't always treated with respect. "I just think that people should educate their nurses more on disabilities and to see that it [doesn't mean] handicapped [necessarily]. It doesn't mean you have to stay home . . . because you've got a disability; you can still work."

Nurse educators and administrators should take the lead and not only educate students but their colleagues, peers, and employees so that we can increase awareness and thereby garner support for our colleagues with disabilities.

> Making organizations aware, that would probably be the best thing. It starts with education, right? Letting organizations know that you can have a physical disability and your job would be completely unaffected but how much better you could do at work if you had the tools at your job. . . . It's very difficult to know that [in] nursing, I don't think we are as friendly to handicaps as we need to be.

A far more sweeping change in nursing education would involve actively encouraging academically and otherwise qualified applicants with physical and/or sensory disabilities to apply to nursing programs throughout the country. Typically, nursing programs are not receptive to students who cannot walk quickly, lift or otherwise do the physical care required in nursing clinical courses. How many intelligent critical thinkers are we potentially losing from the profession? One nurse in a wheelchair described her positive experience in nursing school:

> They gave me the accommodations that I needed. I had a person who was my accommodation . . . who helped me change beds and lift up patients and put bed pans in. I mean, if I can verbalize how to do something, it's the same as actually doing it when you're thinking about competency right? [If] I am knowledgeable enough to know how to instruct someone to do it, [isn't that] the same as . . . actually doing it yourself in a sense? That's what my school had decided, you know—equal.

This nurse had the same clinical training as everyone else, since the school provided assistants to aid her while she was a student.

> The people who helped me did get a small amount of money to help me, but [they] were doing it because they wanted more experience, too. I had a physical therapy student who followed me around so she was getting experience herself, as well as taking care of patients firsthand. [The school] paid for that.

The physical therapy student not only got to provide hands-on care to patients, but also learned how to work with the disabled by assisting the student nurse. What a terrific and very workable idea!

One nurse educator who was interviewed pondered why nurses with disabilities aren't more readily accepted:

> I often wonder about nurses who are blind and I waited for us to get some students who are handicapped in more ways than we are seeing yet, that really require a lot of accommodations and they never seem to turn up. It is interesting. I am not sure how that happens. We get people with mental health issues which are more subtle and more difficult to pick up until people are under a lot of stress. We have had a lot of students in that situation. Rarely [have we] had handicapped students. . . . I don't think there are really any role models. I don't think we put much into that.

Acting as role models is what educators do and it is imperative that nurse educators provide an example of collegial behavior and *esprit d'corps*. It is concerning that we can accept and retain students with mental health problems who may potentially be unsafe with their peers and patients, but cannot see our way to admitting and retaining students with physical disabilities.

Revamping How We Educate Nurses

> I do think it would be worthwhile to explore more the whole shame and silence that goes along with disability and the disabled nurse.... There is something so very isolating about the experience of becoming disabled and that initial reaction of the health care community and that [is the] really important nexus where we can decide that interventions at that particular time can keep the person in practice or truly create an almost psychosocial barrier that an individual may never overcome.... I think you can either have in the faculty setting faculty who are just deathly afraid of working with the student because of the potential liability for them and I guess their focus can be on themselves or you can have faculty who are very focused on helping that student navigate that process. [I had] a faculty for my senior practicum ... [who was a] woman [who] had extraordinary courage, wanting to take me on and to have to deal with some of the reactions that came up and she did so and it was her and faculty like her that enabled me to become an RN and I even graduated with the award from my class for excellence in clinical practice. (Neal-Boylan & Guillett, 2008)

One possible alternative to the current educational system is to have all nursing students take the same generalist courses, such as fundamentals of nursing, medical-surgical nursing, obstetrics, pediatrics, and mental health nursing but provide nursing students with disabilities with different clinical experiences. In other words, the student with a disability might have a clinical experience at a pediatric private practice rather than at a hospital or might work with a nurse case manager instead of on a medical-surgical floor (Box 8.1).

Alternatively, the student with a disability might observe clinical practice in the same sites as other students. They could still plan care but would delegate any physical work that they were unable to do. For example, a student in a wheelchair could still care for patients on the hospital

---

Box 8.1 Student With a Disability Has Alternative Clinical Courses

- Student takes all of the nursing theory/didactic courses that all of the other students take
- Student is assigned alternative clinical experiences, such as informatics, school nursing, research, case management, education, etc.

Might require a limited license

floor but could plan the care and delegate the physical work, most likely to a nurse's aide. Physicians with disabilities, just like able-bodied physicians, delegate a lot of work to nurses. A visually impaired student could be paired with an aide or perhaps another student to carry out the clinical work required. Perhaps, as in the example given earlier, a physical therapy or occupational therapy student could be paired with a nursing student who has a disability. They could learn from each other.

Hearing-impaired students are typically limited by those around them failing to speak directly to them or by the lack of assistive devices on phones. This could be easily remedied by paying closer attention to the student's needs.

One nurse practitioner who uses a wheelchair described how she cares for her patients even though she has physical limitations:

> I was taking care of a patient not too long ago. She was elderly . . . and she had fallen. She was lying on a stretcher and she had fallen and hit her hip and I needed to do range of motion on her hip but because she was on a stretcher, it was too high for me to reach so I had one of the nurses come over and I told her how to check for range of motion and how to move her leg in such a way and to feel for certain things and then watch [the patient's] face and see if she's cringing and if there's cramping, things like that, so we could get that element of the exam done even though I didn't physically do it.

The student would then be assigned to specific clinical experiences in areas of nursing that do not require physical strength. The student could work with a case manager, a research nurse, an informatics nurse, or a nurse in another area (Box 8.2). For example, a student who plans to go into school nursing could receive clinical experiences specific to that role.

Box 8.2 Student With a Disability Has a Mix of Observational and Hands-On Clinical Experiences

- Student takes all of the nursing theory/didactic courses that all of the other students take
- Student observes in the clinical settings in which he or she is physically unable to perform the skills
- The student is provided with a variety of experiences that she or he is physically able to do, such as school nursing, advice nursing, case management nursing, etc.

Student should receive same license as other graduates

This would also provide an opportunity to educate students about all of the different types of nursing jobs there are.

It is interesting to consider why hospital care is the primary focus of clinical practica when so much care is provided in community settings. Even if nursing curricula and practica were to remain as they are now, why couldn't a student with a disability take all of the same courses with other students, but perform a more observant role in clinical practicum settings that have a lot of physical requirements and take a more active role in clinical settings that don't require as much physical work?

A student who plans to go into informatics could work with a nurse who is employed in that position. One nurse with a disability who works in an informatics position had this to say:

> I knew . . . for a long time that I really enjoyed the IT (information technology) field and that I would be interested in blending my nursing skills with the IT field and that's about the time that . . . positions started opening. . . . People were starting to make a move toward electronic charting anyway and that was starting to open up these positions. . . . I found a job and actually we relocated for me to take a job in that field. . . . There's a very high demand for people in this position. It's worked out ideally for me. You don't need actually an IT background to go into it. What they look for is just more of a nursing background for the type of position I'm in because they can teach you what you need to know about computers but they can't teach you nursing education. They can't take an IT person and teach them everything they need to know about nursing to do the job effectively. It's very much a growing field.

The student who cannot do the physical work of the hospital could still plan and supervise the patient's care, but delegate the physical work. Having a physical disability should not prevent the student from being able to understand what his or her patient needs, design a realistic and sensible plan of care, or be able to show empathy to patients. In general, it would seem that nurses with illnesses or disabilities are more likely to be empathetic than those who are well and able-bodied. One nurse with a disability said: "I had had empathy but I really, really in my heart, felt empathy for my patients after I got sick."

In certain other countries, the United Kingdom, for instance, student nurses enroll in school in a specific track that is available because the National Health Service deems that there is a shortage of nurses in a particular area. For instance, a student may enter nursing school specifically to be prepared as a nephrology or a cardiac nurse. Nursing schools in the United States could emulate this example by admitting nursing students into various tracks at the start. All nursing students, regardless of whether they have a disability, would be admitted into a particular track. Courses and clincials experiences would be assigned depending on the track the student had chosen (Box 8.3).

This alternative would work quite well for students with disabilities and might, in fact, be appreciated by any student who attends nursing school with the intention of working in a specialty nursing practice. This idea might also help prevent and/or manage future nursing shortages.

Students who are unable to walk might be trained to be advice nurses or to work in informatics among other possibilities. A visually impaired student might train to be a case manager and be able to use assistive technology to do the job.

Student nurses with disabilities might think it unfair that they are singled out by having alternative clinical experiences. In that case, it might benefit all nursing students to have a general curriculum that is followed by a specialized curriculum (Box 8.4). This is standard practice in Master's in Nursing programs. Students take a certain number of core courses and then branch off into their specialty areas by taking specialized courses and participating in practica for these specialties. A new graduate nurse might then receive a limited license based on his or her specialty area.

This may seem a foreign and distasteful concept to some, but physicians have been doing it for a very long time as have nurses in other

---

Box 8.3 All Nursing Students Enter School in a Predetermined Track

- All nursing students enter the nursing program in a predetermined track.
- Clinical experiences are tailored according to each track, such as inpatient hospital, long-term care, community/public health, case management, research, etc.

Will require a limited license

Box 8.4 All Nurses Receive a Generalist Foundation With Specialty Tracks

- All students receive didactic and theory courses in generalist subject areas, such as obstetrics, pediatrics, medical-surgical nursing, and mental health.
- Each student chooses a specialty track to continue their education.

Would require a specialty license

countries. Rather than exclude bright, capable prospective students from entering nursing programs, might it be possible to offer the option of a limited license as opposed to a generalist license such as we now provide?

The increasing use of simulation in nursing education could allow the student with a disability to practice skills in the lab using assistive devices or a person to aid them. They could then get checked off on the skills, but not be expected to perform them on live patients if the student is not considered to be able to do that safely. Different jobs and settings require different skills. This author recently heard of a nursing student with a disability who was otherwise doing well in class and in her clinical experiences, but could not catheterize a patient due to her disability. The school was considering failing this student in the course. Yet, after this student becomes a registered nurse, she may never have to catheterize a patient. Should she be dismissed from the course and probably the program simply because she cannot manage this skill? No, she should be shown how to do the skill in the lab or observe others performing it in the clinical setting. She should perform the skills as best she can in the lab and be evaluated in terms of passing the course on whether she understands why we might catheterize a particular patient, and the contraindications and complications associated with catheterization. When she applies for a job or gets one, she will then be faced with needing to perform the skills required for the position. This nurse will need to explain that she cannot catheterize a patient and it will then be up to the nurse manager to determine whether or not this disqualifies her from the job.

Nurse educators and administrators should role model acceptance and understanding of people with disabilities and not be so quick to discard potential or current students who might make great nurses because they are unable to do everything other students can. It is important to creatively explore what else the nursing student with disabilities might be able to do to demonstrate his or her ability to become a great nurse.

Suggestions for the Student With a Disability

> I think from the perspective of a nursing school, you really have to support students but [they] also have to have accountability around making sure the combination (of clinical experiences) [the students] need [is] available and then that they are really comfortable talking about what they need, to be successful and safe in a situation.

Nursing students with disabilities who are currently in nursing school programs should be made aware of their rights and resources when they are accepted into school and should be reminded of these throughout their stay in school. This information should be provided to all nursing students as anyone might have a hidden disability or develop a disability while in school. Students should make their disabilities known to their advisors and faculty, and describe their needs for accommodation. The student disability center on each campus will evaluate the student and give them official permission to receive accommodations.

> When I was told by my advisor if you don't apply to the department of disabilities, we cannot accommodate anything, we cannot think of accommodations, [I was] torn apart. My husband actually went online to the university's webpage and looked at that part of the webpage for the disability office and it actually says that it is the student's responsibility to decide to contact that office and to do the application for that office and that the professors actually are not supposed to suggest it to anybody because it might be construed as being prejudiced against them. . . . I think it is ridiculous that nobody suggested it because clearly I didn't know that was an option for me. I didn't think of myself as being disabled. I didn't know that they would accept students who just had a temporary problem. I had no clue at all. This was a new thing for me.

Prospective and current students should critically evaluate whether or not they think they have a disability and, if they are unsure, to inquire at the school's student disability center. If the student knows that he or she has a physical or learning disability it behooves him or her to acknowledge this up front and ask for an assessment by this office. A note from a health care provider is typically not sufficient to get accommodations for such students.

If the student does not acknowledge the disability and consequently fails all or part of a course, faculty will rarely be willing to change a grade to accommodate a disability that was never revealed. Faculty are obligated to do all they can to protect the student's confidentiality by not singling them out because they have a disability, but cannot do anything if they are unaware of the disability. Moreover, faculty are not supposed to ask a student directly if they are disabled so students should not expect this.

Suggestions for the Faculty With a Disability

It is important that nursing faculty with disabilities also receive reasonable accommodation as required by law, and not be shunned or isolated by their peers. Deans and department Chairs should be cognizant of the necessary accommodations and assign courses and classrooms based on each faculty's nursing expertise and physical abilities. Why must a nurse with mobility problems teach in an amphitheater? Why can't a nurse with the necessary expertise teach a clinical course or a skills lab if others are available to do the physical work and demonstrations? An honest effort should be made to sit down with the faculty member and discuss the accommodations that might be required so that the nursing program can take full advantage of the faculty's expertise. As mentioned earlier, it might be possible for a nurse with disabilities to teach or demonstrate skills via simulation in a more manageable way than in the actual clinical setting.

EMPLOYMENT

There is, unfortunately, a public perception or public opinion of nurse's jobs as being very physical even though when you look today, a lot of nurse's aides, patient care assistants are doing a lot of the physical work. There is still that kind of traditional idea and it's hard for people to see that a person can be a nurse and not be able to do those physical things. What we need to do is reframe the idea of nursing. What is nursing? Is nursing about assessment and evaluation and planning, which are skills that you develop through knowledge? Or is it about making beds and changing diapers and lifting up patients? Is that what nursing is because if we make that the limiting factor then we're basically [saying] that's who we are and that's what it is. We can't make that the limiting factor in terms of who can do the job and not do the job.

This book has illustrated the many ways in which nurses with disabilities have been treated differently from their peers and colleagues for reasons related to their disability. Reducing and eliminating discrimination begins with the hiring process. Nurses who present for an interview should be viewed for potential employment based on their nursing qualifications, not their physical attributes.

Research indicates that in some ways nurses with visible disabilities fare better than those with "invisible disabilities" because it is clear to see what accommodations they might need and they are often provided with them. However, other nurses with visible disabilities never hear back about whether or not they got the job after being interviewed, and are not likely to have discussions with nurse recruiters or managers about what they can or cannot do given their particular disability.

Embrace the nurse that has disabilities and let her do what she can do and just keep going with it . . . Embrace what they[ve] got instead of [looking at] what the person can't do. It just doesn't make sense to me to just do that. It's just totally ridiculous to abandon, throw them out when they could still make a contribution to the human race.

Nurses most often hid their disabilities if it was possible to do so because they feared or had learned from experience that they might not get a job if they revealed their disabilities, and they were prepared to do whatever it took to meet its requirements. A study on whether nurses with disabilities' job descriptions actually matched the work required found that when nurses were given job descriptions (which didn't always occur) they were generally able to do what was asked. It was more often things that were not listed on the job description that caused supervisors and colleagues to find fault with the nurse. For example, a nurse might be expected to lift or move a patient even if that was not listed on the job description.

The ideal situation would be for the nurse with a disability, whether it is visible or invisible, to feel comfortable revealing the disability or chronic illness to the recruiter or nurse manager without fear of losing the job or of other repercussions. According to the law, a nurse recruiter must be certain that a disabled applicant actually cannot do what is expected in the job. Simply making an assumption because the applicant walks with a cane or gets up from a chair slowly is not enough. Many of the nurses studied said they would have been willing to demonstrate skills or tasks that were in doubt rather than to have lost a job. Since many organizations require that the employee pass a physical exam prior to being hired any "red flag" regarding health issues should be identified and discussed at that time as well.

As things presently stand, it is hard to recommend to nurses with disabilities that they be open and forthright regarding their disability in a job interview because there are still nurse recruiters and managers who may be inclined to have pre-conceived ideas about what nurses with disabilities can do. It may be hoped, however, that in the future nurses with disabilities will be able to speak openly about what they are unable to do and feel confident that if they do not have the capability to perform a particular job they will be directed to another job that they can do. Certainly, we should hope they will not be dismissed out of hand before having the opportunity to demonstrate what they have to offer.

Most of the nurses studied readily agreed that they couldn't work in every job and viewed what was best for the patient as paramount. Yet they felt excluded from jobs they could safely do, often with little individual consideration given to their particular expertise or abilities. One nurse with rheumatoid arthritis shared some specific methods she uses to be able to perform her critical care job.

> If [I have to] empty a Foley [catheter], I slide the chair over, sit down in the chair, empty the Foley. I never scooch down. I can't scooch down, I have bad knees. I bend at the waist. I put the bed up high when I'm doing vital signs, put the bed down when I'm done.... When [patients] void [they] always [have] those little stands that you put in front of the bed for the patient to put their feet down on first and then they come down because the beds are so high sometimes.... When I'm helping with a Swan [Ganz], I put one leg up on [the stand] because it helps my back.... There was this morning that we put in a Swan, vented somebody and we did an A[rterial] line. I was in there a good 4½ hours and I did alright until right to the end of it when the doc said something to me about doing some other thing. I said "Just a minute, could we take a little break?" I just needed to get off my feet for a second.... The other nurse said she'd go in and do it 'cause everything was set up but the doctor said he would rather that [I do it]. I said, "But I can't right now." So I'm good at ICU. I know what I'm doing. I know how to take care of my patients.... It just shows me how foolish some nurses can be about what they think, because another nurse is thinking that [I'm] deliberately trying to get out of doing something, [which] is ridiculous. It's just totally ridiculous. Why would you go to work if you don't want to do it?

This nurse's story illustrates that not only could she do her job with minor compensatory techniques but that her skills were sought after by the physician regardless of her disability. Nevertheless, other nurses thought that she might be trying to get out of doing her work when she needed time to take a break.

Reasonable Accommodation

> There is so much that nursing can offer. There is so much.... We take care of patients with disabilities and we don't look at them for their disabilities. We look at what they are able to do and you have resources for patients so why not for nurses who take care of patients?

Those nurses who are hired should receive reasonable accommodation as described in Chapter 1. They should not have to fight to get the equipment they need to help them to perform their jobs. Among other things, nurses who are given desk jobs should be given the right desk, computer, and telephone that allow them to be safe ergonomically. Hearing-impaired nurses should have phones equipped with assistive devices and not have to worry that others will tamper with or remove them. Managers should ensure that hearing-impaired nurses get written reports of any information that is provided verbally to staff. One nurse suggested that instead of or in addition to audible alarms "a flashing light so if I can't hear it, at least I can see it." This nurse also said that the organization should be able to provide stethoscopes for the hearing impaired. Visually impaired nurses should be provided with information in Braille and computer technology that will enable them to work.

Nurses who qualify for handicapped parking should be granted those privileges and the setting in which they work should be consistent with their need for easy access. For example, a nurse who qualifies for a handicapped parking place should also have an ergonomic work station that is likewise easily accessible. One nurse manager commented:

> We make sure that passageways and doorways are wide enough and the entrance is accessible. There's a chair bathroom, but certainly the attitudes in this place are, I believe, open and accepting and inclusive so if a person with disabilities would interview for a position, I do not believe there would be any resistance.

A nurse who has trouble lifting patients because of a disability might be assigned patients who can move themselves, lighter patients, or an aide that can partner with the nurse. One nurse explained that even though her job description for her home care position required heavy lifting, she was able to get an accommodation.

> It's some place [on the job description that] there's a weight limit. I believe you're supposed to be able to lift 50 pounds but because I'm not full time . . . if I say what kind of patient is it and they say it's a bed-ridden 300-pound patient, I say I don't think I can do to that one. So I am able to choose where I go.

Job Descriptions

> There is a crying need for nurses. I almost think hiring a nurse with a disability would be a good selling point for the hospital or the facility by marketing equal opportunity employment . . . especially if there are some desk jobs and phone calls and online things like crisis hotlines or doctor's offices. There are all kinds of [jobs].

Job descriptions should be carefully crafted to list the actual work required and nurses with disabilities should not be penalized when they cannot do something that is not specified on the job description. Managers and administrators should consider whether their staff really need to lift 50 pounds or if others can do that for them. When hiring for a job, the nurse's expertise, background, and ability to think critically should be given utmost consideration. Are there any physical responsibilities that the nurse can delegate? Is there any task a nurse with a disability can trade to a physically able nurse and do something else in return? Seeing to the needs of patients and clients is the goal. Is there more than one way in which a particular task can be done? As one nurse with a disability lamented:

> I guess there is a severe concern and perhaps an overreaction about the potential risk of hiring a person with a disability. I think that many organizations are unable to look beyond the skill set that an individual brings. They are truly viewed totally and solely in terms of their disability and the potential liability that it might bring and that is such a tragedy. (Neal-Boylan & Guillett, 2008)

The issue of nurse heroics, discussed in Chapter 7, is worth revisiting. All nurses are at risk of burnout, fatigue, and of leaving the profession as a result. Managers, administrators, and nurses in general must respect each other's need to take days off and sick days, and not have to justify why they cannot work those days or work overtime. Nurses should be encouraged to take their breaks and to eat their meals. If they do not care for their own health then they will burn out more quickly and are also at risk of developing illness or disability. It does the organization no good to lose good nurses because they are constantly overworked.

It also does the nursing profession no good to foster an image that nurses don't need rest or sleep or food, and that the organizations that employ nurses should not have to hire enough staff to permit everyone to take their breaks and vacations. Several nurses spoke to the fact that their managers, supervisors, and fellow faculty "work themselves to death," which is not good role modeling for nurses either individually or collectively. "Maybe that makes it self-perpetuating that we look around us and see other nurses doing this so we expect that we should be able to do it."

Perhaps the nurse with a disability can work 4-hour shifts or split 4-hour shifts. Is there a creative way to schedule the work so no one feels overloaded and becomes burned out but all are able to stay on the job? Is there any flexibility regarding how the job is designed?

> I think time flexibility would be the most important thing. Maybe they could be more open-minded as far as looking at your background and saying "You know what? You have a lot to offer.

We realize you can't do the physical work in the traditional sense, work on the floor but . . . we think you would be very helpful in this department, in this situation." Maybe focus more, instead of the physical, more on the interpersonal.

Alternatives

The facility should attempt to accommodate disabled nurses and work with them to find out what it is that they can do, instead of emphasizing what they can't do. When nurses cannot do certain jobs due to their disabilities, administrators and Human Resources personnel should provide information on nursing positions within the organization that would fit with the nurse's skills and abilities. "No one ever sat down and said 'I can see at a distance as an experienced employer [that] you are facing situations here and maybe there are some options you haven't thought of yet.'"

A nurse manager explained:

> I have been asked on occasion to evaluate or rather help locate a nurse who can no longer stay in her department. For example, we had a nurse who worked in the ER who had knee replacement surgery and certainly the job skills required squatting and pivoting and lifting heavy weights . . . but we were able to relocate her in the nursery where the physical requirements were less demanding. . . . We focus on skills and abilities.

Another suggested:

> . . . a task force within an organization with people from all disciplines to look at what's available for possible light duty positions and have that resource available. . . . People with light duty requirements have their case reviewed . . . just look at the disability issue and then come up with a plan.

Some interviewees suggested developing databases that would store information about nursing jobs and their requirements and locations. These databases could be sponsored by national nursing organizations, nurse specialty organizations, and/or within health care agencies. A nurse with a chronic illness or disability could search the database for available jobs by plugging in his or her physical limitations, educational background, expertise, and geographical location. Jobs that would fit the nurse's specifications would then be listed. In this way, nurses would no longer feel the need to leave the profession because they don't know where to find a place that would hire them. A nurse with a disability commented:

> I really think it's important. If for some reason, I wasn't able to do this job, I would hope that my employer would have options available to me and if it wasn't within my facility that they'd at least give me ideas of someplace else or some other contacts where I could still have a career as a nurse.

Another nurse manager explained:

> If you have someone with a lot of experience who can direct the care and is not directly responsible for the hands on but [is] responsible to see that the hands on [care] is done in a way that is reasonable, that is the perfect job for someone who has a physical kind of disability.... I know that the [clinical] nurse leader position would be for someone who directed care for a patient across the health care agency so that as the patient moved through the agency this person moved with the patient. Now that might require additional education but it would be easily accommodated. I don't know about other kinds of disabilities but I do know that there are all kinds [of] assistive devices that could help people and hopefully they'll be used more often in the [inpatient] setting.

When a nurse does have to leave the organization, he or she should receive counseling from the Human Resources department regarding transitioning from one role to another, and managers should give solid references that speak to what the nurse can do on the job, rather than what they can't. One nurse with a disability discussed the "ideal job" she found working in health care informatics.

> I've been a big advocate of people who are looking for nurses that have disabilities to really look into this type of a role. What's evolving is kind of two different roles for nurses. They're kind of split.... You've got the nurses who do [what] I do—mainly support and building up the system—which probably [includes] people who have a higher interest in IT (information technology) work, but then the other world that's developing is what they call "informatics." For me, the traditional nursing informatics role, 15 years ago was definitely more of a data collection type of role. Now, ... nursing informatics is more of a role for nurses who may even do work clinically or at least work at the clinic, the active clinician. [They work on] some of the issues that aren't working

for them when they do their charting, help with the education portion, and they're the ones who will figure out what they need from charting and bring it to the nurses in IT and say we need these changes to the [computer] screen because this isn't working—workflow. Then they take over, do the training on these systems or [train the] employees . . . so it's kind of splitting into two roles which . . . [for] somebody who's not interested in computers but is interested in a similar type of role, that is an opportunity for them to be that liaison between the nurses and the IT department.

Another interviewee discussed seeking and obtaining a desk job that was unaffected by her disability: "This job is basically a desk job. I have patient contact over the phone. I'm sitting at a desk all day so there's no problem with my ankle at all." This nurse had originally asked for a desk job but was refused "They told me no. I was welcome to come back when I was able to walk again." She had to fight to get her current job. Sometimes taking a chance on a nurse with a disability can benefit both him or her and the hiring organization. Another interviewee said: "The home care people took a chance on me and that was a good thing."

One of the nurses interviewed discussed working in an outpatient oncology clinic. She is an amputee, but this does not impact her ability to use her oncology expertise and experience to care for patients. Unlike previous inpatient oncology positions, her current job description does not require being able to lift 50 pounds.

These patients [may] come in ambulating . . . if they're older . . . they might be on a cane or a walker. Some of them come in on a wheelchair with their care provider. . . . I did help the other day with someone who had a really hard time getting out of the chair and we used good body mechanics, lifting technique. We were on each side and just helped him to stand and it really wasn't that demanding having shared the load with somebody. . . . There really isn't much [that's physical] in this setting, which I am grateful for.

A nurse manager agreed:

[An] ambulatory care center [would be good for a nurse with a disability]. It's very unlikely that there's time sensitivity. We may have productivity issues but time sensitivity, probably not, safety probably not. People are coming in for allergy shots, pre-op[erative] testing. It's different. What it will take is a thorough consideration of what types of positions could be accommodated and aggressively seeking to do just that.

Another interviewee suggested that nurses with disabilities have first call for jobs that do not require physical work.

> I've been thinking that although I can qualify for what we used to call cushy jobs in these offices, 9 to 5, I don't care about the hours, I could work at night ... but most of these positions in nursing where they do paperwork, evaluations, and that sort of thing are done by people who have all of their capacities, all of their senses, and they're healthy. I think that maybe if they would require ... hiring the disabled first like someone who can't hear who doesn't have to hear to do paperwork ... have disabled first do those jobs. ... There's no real open door for the people with disabilities to get into nursing to do things that they could do, that very capable nurses who are physically able to do are now offered.

A nurse manager described how a nurse with a permanent injury was given other responsibilities so the organization could keep her.

> She had this limp so actually running up and down the hall taking care of the patient just wasn't going to work out for her anymore. So, ... she was on special projects. She sorta turned into the quality assurance, infection control [person]. We gave her responsibilities that required her to use her nursing brain not her nursing back, a job [in which] she could stand up and sit down. I think we actually got her back 2 hours a day to start. She'd stay 2 hours and then she'd go. I think she's still here. She works full time and she takes care of those things.

This manager shared other suggestions regarding nurses with disabilities.

> We have those centers now where you call in and talk to a nurse over the phone so I could envision somebody who was having trouble walking or even using their arms, being able to use their brain and talk to people. [In a long term care facility] there's a 14-page assessment tool. Every admission results in 3 hours of paperwork. And the first part is the Minimum Data Set (MDS) and it's a specialty. The manual is 600 pages long. ... The evening supervisor is responsible for trying to get the majority of the paperwork done ... and it's because she has a condition with her hip that causes a great deal of pain and being a clinical nurse was getting to be torture for her, [that] we created this other position (MDS nurse) and she did well. ... My job is to put in place whatever I could put in place to help those people do their jobs. I am

proud of us for figuring out [a way to] take care of that nurse to our own advantage. It's worked great by the way. We have higher quality MDS than we've ever had.

A management job is worth considering for a nurse with a disability if he or she meets the necessary qualifications. A recruiter had this suggestion:

A person who had a physical disability, if they have the qualifications, could probably be a person in a management role. I don't see them as being particularly able to do hands on care particularly . . . but as far as mental agility, that person certainly could be capable of managing a unit as long as they had the education and training behind them.

Other nurse recruiters and managers echoed this thought and also suggested case manager, quality manager, educator, and researcher as positions that could be done without physical effort. "There are research positions and quality improvement teams and education . . . and we have case managers." One manager commented:

In my facility, we did use LPNs (licensed practical nurses) in our telemetry unit secretary role because they were also able to take orders from physicians which was really nice to be able to do. If you had a crisis and you had RNs actually tied up in a room, you still had somebody who could answer phones, read the scrips, and be able to speak to the physician and take orders, so that was a nice role. . . . If we could figure out a way to use the knowledge everyone has, that certainly would be to our advantage.

Some nurse recruiters and managers gave specific ideas about what a nurse with a disability could do to remain in nursing:

We have a nurse who's in a risk management position. We have nurses who oversee managed care and utilization review, so they're not as directly involved in patient care but very critical roles within the hospital. . . . Staff development [is another possible role].

Another nurse manager described how it could be helpful to have a nurse with an illness or disability take over some of the committee work and other tasks required of nurses.

We want very much for staff registered nurses to be involved in shared governance and quality improvement and committee

> work, etc. So, if you can't spare the young healthy people from the bedside, okay, this is the perfect job [for someone with a disability]. We have a nurse upstairs who has cancer and she is operating under the regular job descriptions and she gets full assignments but we have kind of selected her to be our committee guru. Whenever there is someone who needs to be on a committee or be selected on a team, we pick her because we know it is better for her.

ON THE JOB

> Because someone's in a wheelchair doesn't mean that [they] can't do this and this. If someone has a fatigue problem, maybe they can work 2 days a week and then don't try to make them feel guilty. There is a lot of guilt in nursing right now, too much guilt about you really have to stay and get this done. People aren't motivated by guilt, they're motivated by doing a good job and being rewarded for that and . . . [nursing should] not use people and overextend them.

Once the nurse with a disability is on the job, it is important that he or she is treated respectfully. Administrators and managers should set the tone by treating everyone fairly, and should not tolerate hurtful teasing or isolation of nurses who are different in some way. Nurses who cannot work above and beyond the job description or who must use all of their sick days should not be labeled as shirkers or malingerers. Certainly a manager should not—as one nurse described earlier in this book—call a meeting in which nursing staff are encouraged to ventilate about how they feel about working with a disabled colleague. This is akin to calling such a meeting to discuss working with a person of another color or ethnicity, which would rightly be deemed unconscionable.

> I have found that in 30 years of nursing, nurses, on the whole, eat their young. I really believe that and it makes me sick. . . . I won't have it, one comment [about] back stabbing or bitchiness. . . . That's how I ran my staff when I was supervising or charge nurse. Good Lord, life is tough enough, you need to come to work and do your work and then go home. . . . We are role models and should be role models . . . . I think mentoring and role modeling are wonderful. . . . If we see one of our brothers or sisters in our profession in need, we should be proactive. That would be wonderful.

Administrators and managers should not make assumptions about what nurses with disabilities can and cannot do, but should instead ask them. There also needs to be an environment of acceptance and understanding, and of believing that nurses with disabilities *can* do their jobs until proven otherwise. One nurse practitioner remarked on the benefits of such an environment:

> It's been wonderful. The patients have been really great and the nurses have been great as well. I don't think any of my requests related to my disability have been received in a not-right way. Sometimes there are assumptions made like maybe she can't do this but they always ask, which is good. They'll say do you think this is a good patient for you to see or do you think somebody else should see this patient? They might say, "Hey this patient's already got a wheelchair and a stroller in the exam room. It will probably be hard for you to get around, do you want me to pass this patient to someone else?" . . . That's something I'm reasonable with where another person can take care of that and I can take care of someone else. I don't think people or the nurses see me as any less because of that, that I can't take care of those kinds of patients because they know it's not because of my competence, it's because of the space.

This nurse practitioner went on to describe her struggle to find a job in which others would be supportive, and suggested that nurses with disabilities work to change the minds of people who don't know what is possible for them.

> In general, I can usually change people's minds. . . . People have a preconceived notion of what nursing is and if they see me in action all of a sudden it makes sense to them, how this works. It's hard for people to imagine things that they've never considered before.

A nurse manager discussed how a nurse practitioner in her hospital was able to work despite a disability.

> We have a nurse practitioner who has MS (multiple sclerosis) and she has a scooter and we were delighted to hire her. Her scooter requirements are for any long distance walking but in terms of provision of care in our contained NICU (neonatal intensive care unit), she is more than able to navigate, ambulate when she needs to. So, here was a case where she wanted to work in the NICU. It is a contained unit. The requirements for her scooter were limited. It had no intrusion in her job role which is a little bit different than the registered nurse, so it was a no brainer, no problem.

Suggestions for the Nurse Recruiter or Administrator

> I think the clinical agencies are going to have to work to figure out how to protect people with disabilities. There are tremendous vacancies all over the place and ... the kind of nursing that is practiced in the clinical setting has to change to accommodate all kinds of people. I think it's probably easily done by using ancillary staff in other kinds of positions.

Follow the Law and Agency Policy
Administrators should be careful that existing policies and rules are followed. For example, to accommodate nurses with severe allergies, some facilities have policies against staff wearing perfumes, scented soaps, and cosmetics. These policies are not always followed, to the detriment of the nurses, patients, and their families.

All nurses should receive regular notification of their disability and Family Medical Leave Act rights and options. A nurse should not have to leave a job because he or she is unaware of their legal rights. Providing this information at orientation is not sufficient.

> If I thought I was better qualified than someone, even with a disability, then [it would be great if] I could go to some board or something and say "Why are they hiring so and so instead of me?" I just don't want to get involved in any disputes about why didn't you hire me or why did you hire that person.

It is up to the administrator, recruiter, or nurse manager to ensure that the nurse with a disability is viewed fairly both when it comes to hiring and while the nurse is on the job. As one nurse manager put it: "I think you really have to look at the individual and their disability. I'm truly amazed by the capabilities that some people with disabilities have and how they have accommodated ... to make up for the disability."

Help Nurses With Disabilities Remain on the Job

A nurse manager gave an example of how a nurse with a hearing impairment remained an effective nurse.

> In my early years of nursing, I did work with a nurse who was very hard of hearing. She had hearing aids in both ears. She didn't use sign language but she relied upon us talking directly to her and she was a very effective nurse. She became an assistant head nurse and she was very effective with patients. Sometimes I think she

kind a slowed down a little bit more in her verbal communication with the patients and maybe presented a less hurried manner which ended up being an asset. Patients really seemed to appreciate her and relate to her.

Another nurse manager spoke of the need to be creative about jobs and who can do them.

We have a lot of nurses that probably could be utilized in positions if we got a little more creative in scheduling, making the work place a little more adaptive than it is. One great concern of mine is that [in] many facilities, a nurse is doing a great job until they get injured and then . . . if you are out on disability for more than 90 days, they eliminate your position stating that you no longer meet the requirements of your job physically. I'm not sure that's always the case. Perhaps employers as nurse manager recruiters should do a little more to make the work place after injury more conducive to . . . a nurse's behavior and skills set so that they can continue to work. We have a lot of investment in RNs and there's a huge nursing shortage as well as the average age of our nurses is like 47 or 48 years old . . . and we need to keep them employed as long as we can for the benefit of the profession.

Appreciate What Nurses Bring to Nursing

In the final analysis, the most important thing is that a nurse knows his or her job and is able to perform it. Yet the attitude that a nurse brings to the workplace is also important, and here nurses with disabilities may have something special to offer. As one nurse manager put it:

I think that hiring someone with a disability can be a very good thing for an organization. I think what I really look for in employees transcends kind of disability. I'm looking for people with the right attitude, people that I believe are going to be respectful to the patients and are truly interested in helping them and . . . are kind and respectful to the patients and I don't think it matters if you are disabled or not. Those are really the attitudes, the essential attitudes, qualities or capabilities I'm looking for in an employee. . . . I value and I have an openness to looking at whomever the individual is that comes in for an interview on a particular day. . . . I also believe that someone who has a disability and you determine that that disability can be accommodated in the particular setting, that they're looking for the job and I think that they can add a tremendous richness to the work place and really inspire people because of what they've been able to do with managing their own disability.

Create and Maintain a Welcome Work Environment

Another nurse manager said that teamwork was the key to allowing everyone to be able to complete their work and also have time to take breaks and manage the workload.

> Everybody helps each other. It's an expectation that when you are in there, nobody's sitting down eating their supper until everybody's caught up. There's a sense of teamwork. I've worked in other units where it was everybody for themselves. You could be [with] your hair standing straight out and nobody would offer to do anything for you. . . . [Here] everything gets done because we all do it. These are all our patients and we've got 12 patients that we're taking care of, not I have these two patients that I'm taking care of and the heck with the rest of the whole place.

Promote Awareness and Understanding of Disability: Dispel Myths

> I would say that we need to develop some sort of guidelines or a code or a disabled health care professional's bill of rights that is posted in workplace settings. I know there are similar documents completed by the ADA (Americans with Disabilities Act) but somehow have fallen short of really addressing the real-life experiences of nurses. I think we need to initiate training programs for HR (Human Resources) personnel to ensure that they are aware but I don't think it can stop with HR. I think it needs to continue down every level of the organization. I think that staff nurses need to be aware that their disabled colleague is welcome in that organization and what the organizational expectations are about ensuring that individual is able to practice safely and effectively and how other RNs can assist in that process.

It seems clear that there is a widespread suspicion that a nurse with disability is likely to provide patient care that is less safe than other nurses would provide. Yet there is no evidence to support this belief, which appears to stem from sheer prejudice. It is not fair to assume that a nurse with a disability is unsafe. Once again, good communication is key. It is important to talk with the nurse one-on-one if there is any concern and to explore in what way the nurse might be unsafe. It may even be necessary for the nurse with a disability to demonstrate a skill about which there is a concern.

However, the fact remains that any nurse can be unsafe for reasons unrelated to having a disability. Thus, one could make the case that all nurses should have to demonstrate that they are safe performing every skill and that nurses with disabilities should not be singled out. Most health care agencies require nurses to "check off" that they are competent in certain skills. Why should the nurse with a disability be treated any differently in this regard?

> There is a level of concern that needs to be dispelled about the fitness of the person for the job. Let me tell you, disabled people know their limits. They know what they can do and cannot do and if they have had the appropriate rehabilitation and education, they know how to behave in any environment.... There is no real evidence to suggest that nurses with disabilities are a liability. I am not aware of any incident involving a disabled nurse that had a poor outcome. It is just a worry that [administrators] have. We need to dispel that worry.

Nurses with disabilities often devise their own methods for compensating when they cannot perform tasks in the traditional way. Nurses should be given an opportunity to demonstrate these methods and show that they are safe and reasonable. Those in the nursing profession, which is both an art and a science, should recognize that there is more than one way to do many nursing tasks. Our increasing emphasis on evidence-based practice attests to the fact that we have been doing many things for years solely because we have always done them that way—and that when these methods are actually tested they don't always turn out to be the best.

Several interviewees mentioned their inability to perform cardiopulmonary resuscitation (CPR) as the reason why they were not hired or were let go from jobs. Being able to do CPR is a realistic requirement. Yet, once again, it is important to evaluate whether a particular nurse must be able to do CPR or if having use of a defibrillator in the case of cardiac arrest would be enough. Must every nurse be assigned to respond to a code situation or might the nurse with a disability cover the other patients while other nurses respond? If a nurse cannot run down a hallway, does that make her ineligible for the job? In some cases the answer will be an unequivocal "yes" but it is not an answer that should be rushed into without careful thought regarding what is really required.

Value Every Nurse

> Acknowledge my skills and that I'm a plus for management and [see that] they [will] lose out terribly when they won't let me work.

Any good organization wants its employees to be good at what they do. If a nurse has the appropriate expertise, knows how to do the job, and is good at it, surely it is worthwhile to do everything reasonably possible to keep him or her in the job, or at the very least, in the organization. All that is required is an investment of time to find out what skills and abilities the nurse has and then analyzing what he or she can do for the organization. For example, one interviewee who worked in home care was unable to care for all types of patients because she was limited physically but "they made the trade-off knowing I won't see everyone but they know [that] when I go out there, I'm gonna do a good job."

Sometimes nurses with a disability might be better nurses because they have had the experience of being in pain or fatigued and unable to do everything they or others would like them to be able to. As one interviewee put it:

> Now I know what it feels like to not feel good and feel helpless and hopeless and be in the medical system. So I get it, I'm able to put myself in a patient's shoes now and relate to them. . . . I'm a darn good nurse and in fact, I've become a better nurse since I've gotten sick.

It is interesting that nurses with disabilities who have found jobs that they can do and in which they are accepted often have supervisors or bosses who are either not nurses, or who are ill or disabled themselves. Yet one should not have to be ill or disabled to empathize with a nurse or student with a disability or chronic illness. These nurses should not have to search for someone like themselves in order to find jobs that will provide environments of acceptance.

People in the position of recruiting, managing, or working with nurses with disabilities must somehow be convinced that such nurses should be given a try and are worth keeping in the profession. As one nurse said: "The mindset has to change. . . . [Administrators] have no framework in which to change. The paradigm does not shift [otherwise]."

The word "disability" appears to have connotations that do not allow for positive thinking with regard to the disabled person. Rather, the word lends itself to pity, possibly empathy, but more likely skepticism. One nurse said:

> I think the biggest thing that would be helpful would be for people not to be afraid of the word disability and to be able to say "I see

that you utilize a crutch. I just want to see is there anything that we could do to make your time here easier." It's like the elephant in the room, no one wants to talk about it.

Another nurse spoke about the organizations in which nurses work and how they should demonstrate value.

What's your goal in running this organization? Who do you want it to be for the good of and does the good include the employees and is that as important as whatever else the organization is doing? . . . When you talk about small family businesses and sort of the ideal picture is where the employees are like family and you accommodate their schedules because you know their lives matter and then you look at bigger organizations, the organization's schedule matters, not anybody else's. So that's a value question.

TO THE NURSE WITH A DISABILITY OR CHRONIC ILLNESS

I really didn't think about managing myself as a disabled person and managing my career that way. I just never got into thinking about it like that and I never got any help with that either. If I had been able in hindsight, I think I could have done [things] differently.

Be Your Own Advocate

The stories and experiences of nurses with disabilities have taught that they are well advised to know their rights and protections under the law. They must be their own advocates as it is unlikely that others will advocate for them. Nurse with disabilities should become assertive and stand up for their rights and emphasize their abilities over their inabilities. Nurses should confront others who are being discriminatory toward them and try to teach recruiters, managers, and their fellow nurses to focus on what they bring to the job and how they might work together to get it done. One nurse with a disability described how important it is to know one's rights.

I'm grateful for the FMLA (Family Medical Leave Act). If I need to go to a doctor, I am grateful for that. Legally, they can't give me any BS if I'm not feeling good that day because I'm covered under FMLA.

The downside, according to this nurse, is that in order to get FMLA, you must reveal your disability and that can draw attention to it "... because [having] a bull's eye on [my] back has added tremendous stress."

Knowing about one's rights and trying to increase others' awareness about what nurses with disabilities can contribute are important to improving the overall mindset about disability. According to one nurse:

> It's not just in nursing. It's a whole mindset throughout the country and ... one of the things that I did was become an activist for disabled people in [my state]. I went on Medicare and found out that I needed to purchase additional health care to cover what Medicare didn't cover and that because I was, quote "disabled," they could charge me a hundred to three hundred times the rate of seniors because, according to actuarial studies, I would use more insurance coverage. This was my area of expertise. I knew insurance. I think this is discrimination. There are no data to support it. It is [an] actuarial prediction. I took on a campaign and started letter writing and bombarded [the state capitol] and got to the point that our current governor appointed a deputy to deal with me because he [got] tired of my letters. So I did research and I found out that ... it's not the case in other states and that other states have changed the law. I forced the General Assembly here in [my state] to change the law in favor of disabled individuals.

If a nurse does need to leave the job for disability-related reasons, she or he should not be afraid or reluctant to explore the benefits of going on disability. Nurses should not suffer in silence, but should do what they can to protect and advocate for themselves even if it makes others unhappy with their choices. However, before taking disability benefits, nurses with disabilities should be more assertive about exploring other options to stay in nursing. They should look for jobs that they can do and work to convince others that they deserve a chance to show that they can do them.

Honestly Evaluate What You Reasonably Can Do and Cannot Do

Nurses with disabilities should be honest with themselves and catalog what they bring to the job and what they honestly feel they can no longer do due to age, illness, or disability. While it seems wrong to have to prove oneself when able-bodied nurses may not have to, the nurse with a disability may have to be prepared to demonstrate what he or she can do and prove that they can do it safely in order to dispel wrongly held notions and prejudices. It is important to recognize that there probably are jobs that one cannot do well due to the illness or disability and it is unfair to colleagues, administrators, and especially to clients to have someone in a position that they know they cannot do well, whatever the reason.

However, it is also important to be tenacious and advocate for oneself to get a job that is appropriate. As one nurse said: "My personality is such that I am very tenacious and I'm very self-motivated and I've never quit anything. I've always been able to obtain my goals." Another nurse discussed how she had become stronger though her experience of being disabled.

> I'm coming out of the cloud in a lot of ways. I'm not so hard on myself. I'm not so depressed now that I'm back working. I feel encouraged. I've become more empowered. I feel like I've gotten feistier. . . . I still have a lot to offer. The fact that I can't run up and down a busy unit and take care of 6,000 patients a day doesn't mean I'm not valuable but I did go through all those [emotions]: angry, sad, an incredible sense of loss. . . .

Critically Evaluate Whether or Not to Reveal the Disability

A nurse manager remarked:

> We don't discriminate but if [the nurse with a disability] passes the physical [exam] and they do qualify for the job, there's no reason for us not to hire a person. Of course they have to be honest when they're filling out information about everything, [that it] is true and correct.

One nurse felt that she did the right thing by being honest about her disability.

> I need this job and I would probably suggest to other people [that] if you have the opportunity to start back part time that might be the way to go but just being up front and realistic, just be honest with your employers and tell them where you are instead of attempt[ing] to get hired and then they find out you can or can't do something. I just think that honesty goes a long way and that, in general, nurses are compassionate people and if they see that you have certain skills or gifts [that] they might be willing to work with you for different adaptations or work with you and your limitations; it's a dialogue, you can't assume things.

This nurse has a visible disability and many nurses who were interviewed felt that having a visible disability is easier to reveal and discuss then an "invisible" one. But in either case, it is essential that the nurse accept who he or she is and what he or she can and cannot do. This nurse continues:

> It's fortunate [that] I kind of just had to come to a place of accepting myself and who I was and the changes that had occurred in my life but seeing that in some ways it made me a stronger, more compassionate person with more empathy for those who are suffering and just trying to show that despite the things I may not be able to do in this position, that I did have a lot to bring to the table and that will be true of even people with invisible illnesses because they know what it's like to struggle. They are going to be that much better of a nurse in my opinion. It's too bad that there is some stigma but I think just being upfront and just embracing who you are and what you're dealing with but knowing what you bring as a positive asset to the organization, that can outweigh that. Your strength and your empathy can outweigh one or two things you may not be able to do and might need assistance or adaptation with.

Another nurse with a visible disability warns of the inevitable discrimination nurses should expect to face if their disability is revealed.

> I would say be very, very prepared for a lot of discrimination. Be prepared for the fight. You're gonna have to fight to get any job, it doesn't really matter. Sometimes even though your résumé says that you graduated from a program or that you have certain skills and all that stuff, people don't believe it. You have to actually prove that you are competent and the only way you can do that is to get them to give you a chance. That's what I usually push for when I'm trying to interview for a job. That's what I would suggest someone push for. I wouldn't say, you need to hire me because I'm this, I'm that. I'd say give me a chance to show you what I can do . . . that I can be an asset to your company, your clinic, that patients will respond to me well.

Consider Returning to School

Nurses with disabilities should consider going back to school regardless of their current level of education. If it is financially reasonable, getting a

TABLE 8.1
Some Positions Held by Nurses With Disabilities

School nurse	Health Services Organization nurse
Home health nurse	
Private duty nurse	Health insurance nurse
Advice nurse	Case manager
Informatics nurse	Research nurse
Outpatient clinic	Nurse educator

TABLE 8.2
Resources for Nurses With Disabilities

Society of Nurses with Disabilities: http://www.nursingwithdisabilities.org/
American Association of People with Disabilities: http://www.aapd.com/
Exceptional Nurse: http://www.exceptionalnurse.com/
National Organization of Nurses with Disabilities (NOND): http://www.nond.org/

higher degree can open new doors and opportunities for the nurse with a disability.

Above all it is important that nurses with disabilities and chronic illnesses not give up on nursing. There are jobs that require knowledgeable nurses and in which having a disability will be irrelevant. If others can't help locate these jobs, search the internet and make contacts. Talk to a "head hunter" or search firm and tell them your needs. Table 8.1 lists jobs that nurses with various kinds of disabilities have been able to perform without discrimination or difficulty. Table 8.2 includes some selected resources for information and assistance.

Become a Survivor

Nurses with disabilities have said that it is important to enjoy life and one's work despite the illness or disability.

> I think the thing we have to do is survivorship. . . . Some [times an] unwanted, unwelcome traumatic experience or a body change [occurs] that forever changes how [we] see the world . . . and some people can transcend that experience and go on to lead a meaningful life with joyful aspects and some people can't. They fall in that crevice in the middle and can't see another daylight. . . . We have to be able to teach survivorship . . . be able to come out the other side as a functional person capable of joy and relationships and everything else. How to teach survivorship? I'm not quite sure.

It's also important to maintain a sense of humor and to try to increase awareness by others through education rather than through intimidation or conveying feelings of hurt or betrayal. The nurses interviewed said that humor, as opposed to confrontation went a long way to helping others understand their concerns, although sometimes confrontation was unavoidable. As one nurse manager described how to best help nurses with disabilities in the work place: "I think raising awareness, empowerment of people with disabilities to claim their rights and to pursue them and not let imaginary obstacles get in their way."

CONCLUSION

This book has attempted to portray what it's like to be a nurse with a physical and/or sensory disability through the eyes of those who know that experience. The nursing profession is urged to listen to their voices and to make changes that would allow nursing to practice what it preaches: Caring, Compassion, Collegiality, and Critical thinking. If we want to be recognized and valued for our professionalism and intelligence and not as subservient or parochial, then we must be more open-minded regarding our colleagues as well as our patients.

Changing the way we educate nurses is one route, changing the way we hire and work with our nurse colleagues is another. Actually caring for ourselves and each other instead of merely saying that what we do is vital, because, as one nurse said, we must remember: *"We are all just a blink away from a disability."*

REFERENCES

Cocca-Bates, K., & Neal-Boylan, L. J. (2011). Retired RNs: Perceptions of volunteering. *Geriatric Nursing, 32*(2), 96-105.

Neal-Boylan, L. J., & Guillett, S. E. (2008). Nurses with disabilities: Can changing our educational system keep them in nursing? *Nurse Educator, 33*(4), 164–167.

Appendix

Below please find some resources that might be useful to people with disabilities. This is by no means a complete list. The author has no attachments to any of the web sites listed. The reader is encouraged to do his or her own research to be sure the information is trustworthy and reliable. The reader should not have to pay to obtain any information pertaining to disabilities.

FOR NURSES WITH DISABILITIES

Society of Nurses With Disabilities
   http://www.nursingwithdisabilities.org

Exceptional Nurse
   http://www.exceptionalnurse.com

National Organization of Nurses With Disabilities (NOND)
   http://www.nond.org

SOCIAL SECURITY ADMINISTRATION

http://www.ssa.gov/disability

http://www.socialsecurity.gov/multilanguage/10701-EN.pdf

Social Security Administration: Children with disabilities
   http://www.ssa.gov/pubs/10026.html

The Red Book: A Summary Guide to Employment Supports for Persons With Disabilities Under the Social Security Disability Insurance and Supplemental Security Income Programs
   http://www.ssa.gov/redbook/eng/main.htm

Social Security Disability Help
    http://www.socialsecurity-disability.org/disability-application-process/federal-court

AMERICANS WITH DISABILITIES ACT

ADA Home Page
    http://www.ada.gov

ADA.gov
    http://www.ada.gov/cguide.htm

EMPLOYMENT

https://www.disability.gov/employment

U.S. Office of Personnel Management: Federal Employment of People With Disabilities
    http://www.opm.gov/disability

American Association of People With Disabilities
    http://www.aapd.com

DISABILITY PROGRAMS AND RIGHTS

Laws.com Government Programs
    http://government-programs.laws.com/disabillity-benefits

American Association of Retired Persons
    aarp.org

National Disability Rights Network
    http://www.napas.org

Disability Rights Advocates
    http://www.dralegal.org

Disability Rights Education and Defense Fund
    http://www.dredf.org

Center for Disability Rights Incorporated
    http://www.cdrnys.org

American Civil Liberties Union
  http://www.aclu.org/disability-rights

The Council for Disability Rights
  http://www.disabilityrights.org/adatoc.htm

U.S. Department of Veterans Affairs
  http://www.vba.va.gov/bln/21/compensation

Cornell University Employment and Disability Institute
  http://www.ilr.cornell.edu/edi

Internal Revenue Service: Tax Benefits for Businesses Who Have Employees With Disabilities
  http://www.irs.gov/businesses/small/article/0,,id=185704,00.html

Index

academic environment, interactions in, 129–134
accommodations, 137–143
   for APN, 138
   reasonable, 4, 8, 15, 26, 121, 122, 128, 139, 156, 176, 179–180
ADA, *See* Americans with Disabilities Act
advanced practice nurses (APN), 73, 85, 117
   accommodations for, 138
   compensations for, 138–139
aging nurses, 6
alternatives, 182–187
Americans with Disabilities Act (ADA), 2, 4, 42, 73, 191
   definition of disability, 2
APN, *See* advanced practice nurses

balance, 156–157
Braille system, 59, 100, 180
breathing disabilities, 29, 33
burnout, 154
   characteristics of, 153
   definition of, 153

cardiopulmonary resuscitation (CPR), 41, 66, 109, 192
   and safety, 110–111
career goals, 64
   changing, 75–81
Centers for Disease Control and Prevention (CDC), 2
certified nurse's aides (CNA), 122, 123
clinical setting, nurse in, 35, 40, 107, 138, 175, 177

CNA, *See* certified nurse's aides
cognitive disabilities, 5, 45, 115
compensation, 114, 137–143
compensatory techniques, 10, 20, 96, 118, 179
contract work, nurses in, 71
CPR, *See* cardiopulmonary resuscitation

diabetes mellitus, 114, 152–153
disabilities
   benefits, 7
   definitions of, 2–5
   hearing, *See* hearing disability
   hiding, *See* hiding disability from recruiters
   promote awareness and understanding of, 191–192
   rate of, 2
   research, 3–5, 11–15, 46, 123, 146, 154, 161, 177
   sensory, 2–6, 19–20, 30
   short-term, 7
   unemployment rate for, 6
   visible, *See* visible disability
Disabilities Rights Commission, 29
discrimination, 1, 8–9, 24, 31, 59, 73, 85, 167, 195, 197
duration of work test, 7

EEOC, *See* Equal Employment Opportunity Commission's
emotions, 31–33
employment, 6–7, 177–179

205

environment
    academic, 129–134
    health care, 119–129

Equal Employment Opportunity
    Commission's (EEOC), 8
    definitions of disability, 4
esprit d'corps, 169
ethical imperative for nurses, 147, 148

fairness, 102
Family and Medical Leave Act
    (FMLA), 7, 189, 194, 195
fatigue, 28, 29
favoritism, 20–21, 84
FMLA, *See* Family and Medical
    Leave Act

handicap, 4, 10, 122, 164, 180
hardiness, characteristics of, 154
health care
    environment, interactions in,
        119–121
    professionals with disabilities, 35
    working conditions, integrative
        model of, 11
hearing
    ability to nursing practice, 39
    disability, 9, 30, 135
        hiring, 46, 50
    impaired
        nurse, 88, 97–99, 179
        students, 172
    loss, traumatic, 31
heroics, nurse, 157–164
    characteristics of, 146
    definition of, 146
    impact of, 156
    notion of, 161
hiding disability, 37–61
    from recruiters, 44
    hearing disability, 46, 50
    during job interviews, 49
    perspective of, 48–59
    solutions, 59–61
home care
    agency, 42, 56

nurses in, 65, 67, 77, 87
    private duty, 57, 63, 65, 66, 77

integrative model of health care
    working conditions, 11
intensive care unit (ICU), 34, 77–81
interactions, patients 134–137

job
    descriptions
        issue of, 42
        of nurses, 180–182
    interviews, disability hiding
        during, 49
    opportunities for nurses, 73
    requirements, 21, 43

leaving nursing
    concern for patient safety, 25–26
    decide to, 23–24
    difficulties in meeting expectations,
        20–22
    due to stamina/energy, 20
    emotions, 31–33
    keeping nurses from, 33–34
    physical demands, 27
    repercussions, 24–25
    treated differently, 22–23
    who is, 26–31
licensed practical nurses (LPNs),
    145, 186
lift patients, 20, 27, 126, 180, 182
    issue of, 42–43
limitations, 86–92, 97
long-term care facility, nurse manager
    working in, 44–45
LPNs, *See* licensed practical nurses

meeting expectations, 20–22
mental disorder, 3
mobility issues, 72

Nightingale, Florence, 150–151
night shifts, 22
nurse administrators, 162
    and educators, 169, 175
    suggestions for, 189

nurse educators, 35, 107, 108, 132–134, 148–149, 152, 162, 168
 and administrators, 169, 175
nurse heroics, 157–164
 characteristics of, 146
 definition of, 146
 impact of, 156
 notion of, 161
nurse leaders, 35, 92, 158, 163–164
nurse managers, 98, 101, 148, 149, 182, 183, 184, 186, 196
 hidden from, 60
 recruiters and, 38, 60
 working in long-term care facility, 44–45
nurse practitioner, 135, 188
nurse recruiters, 33, 98, 178, 186
 hidden from, 44–48, 60
 and managers, 38, 60
 suggestions for, 189
Nurse Work Instability Scale, 13
nursing director, 39–40
nursing education, 168–177
 change in, 169
 simulation in, 175
nursing informatics, 183
nursing programs, 169, 174
nursing students, 174

obesity, 46, 100–101
operating room (OR), 79, 112
options, 104–109
orthopedic nurses, 52, 123
overtime in work, 22, 149, 163, 181

pain, 101–102
patients
 first, 147
 interactions with, 134–137
 nurse practitioner, 135
 perspective of, 115–116
 safety of, 25–26, 95–96, 102, 103, 108, 109, 111–114
people with disabilities, 121, 168
 discrimination, 8–9
 employment, 6–7

 unemployment rate for, 6
 in United States, 2
physical disabilities, 19–20, 41
 barriers to, 40
 hiring, 44
 nurse practitioner with, 135
 person with, 186
physical disorder, 3
physicians, 10
 work life experiences of, 13–14
psychiatric nursing, 41, 56
psychiatric unit, manager work on, 40–41
psychological disorder, 3
pushing oneself (myself), 147, 159

reasonable accommodation, 4, 8, 15, 26, 121, 122, 128, 139, 156, 176, 179–180
recent work test, 7
recruiters, nurse, *See* nurse recruiters
Rehabilitation Act of 1973, 8
repercussions, 24–25
resilience, 74
research, 3–5, 11–15, 46, 123, 146, 154, 161, 177
retention, nurse, 167–199
rights, 4, 24, 90, 121, 175, 194, 195

safety of nurse, 114–115
safety of patients, 25–26, 95–96, 102, 109, 111–114
school, back to, 73
school nurse, 58, 68, 70, 88, 105, 106
school nursing, 106
self-identified disabilities, 5
self-sacrifice
 dedication and, 160
 tradition of, 150–155
sensory disabilities, 12–13, 19–20, 30
short-term disability, 7
Social Security Administration, 7
solutions, 59–61, 161–164
speaking ability for nurse, 39
stamina of nurse, 20, 22
statistics, disability, 2

student nurses with disability, 168, 174
student with disability, 171, 172
  suggestions for, 175–176
survivor, 198–199

traditional nursing, 51
traumatic hearing loss, 31, 80
treated differently, 22–23

undue hardship, 4, 8
unemployment rate for disabilities, 6
United States Census Questions on
  Disability, 13

visible disability, 12–13, 49, 177, 197
Visiting Nurse Association (VNA), 80

visually impaired nurses, 99–100, 180
volunteer work, 71

work
  ability to, 71–73
  environment, creating and
    maintaining, 191
  hours for nurses, 22, 71, 152
  overtime in, 22, 149, 163, 181
  requirements to, 39–44
  volunteer, 71
World Health Organization
  (WHO), 3